FELIX GILLE

WHAT IS PUBLIC TRUST IN THE HEALTH SYSTEM?

Insights into Health Data Use

POLICY PRESS 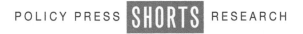 RESEARCH

First published in Great Britain in 2023 by

Policy Press, an imprint of
Bristol University Press
University of Bristol
1–9 Old Park Hill
Bristol
BS2 8BB
UK
t: +44 (0)117 374 6645
e: bup-info@bristol.ac.uk

Details of international sales and distribution partners are available at
policy.bristoluniversitypress.co.uk

The Open Access publication of this book has been published with the support of the
Swiss National Science Foundation.

British Library Cataloguing in Publication Data
A catalogue record for this book is available from the British Library

ISBN 978-1-4473-6733-8 hardcover
ISBN 978-1-4473-6734-5 ePub
ISBN 978-1-4473-6735-2 ePdf

Cover design: Bristol University Press
Front cover image: iStock/a-r-t-i-s-t
Bristol University Press and Policy Press use environmentally
responsible print partners.
Printed and bound in Great Britain by CPI Group (UK) Ltd,
Croydon, CR0 4YY

FSC
www.fsc.org
MIX
Paper | Supporting
responsible forestry
FSC® C013604

Contents

List of figures and tables

Figures

Tables

About the author

Felix Gille is a Postdoctoral Researcher at the Digital Society Initiative, University of Zurich. With a background in European Public Health and Health Policy, Felix currently researches public trust in the context of national electronic health records. Previous publications include: Gille, F. and Brall, C. (2021) 'Limits of data anonymity: Lack of public awareness risks trust in health system activities', *Life Sci Soc Policy*, 17(7). https://doi.org/10.1186/s40504-021-00115-9; Gille, F. and Brall, C. (2021) 'Can we know if donor trust expires? About trust relationships and time in the context of open consent for future data use', *Journal of Medical Ethics*, 48(3). https://doi.org/10.1136/medethics-2020-106244

Acknowledgements

This book covers several years of public trust in the health system research. I started to research public trust for my Master Thesis at Karolinska Institute, Sweden, and at present continue this endeavour at the Digital Society Initiative, University of Zurich, Switzerland. While the main contribution to this book is my 2017 doctoral thesis completed at the London School of Hygiene and Tropical Medicine, England (*Theory and conceptualisation of public trust in the health care system: Three English case studies: Care.data, biobanks and 100,000 Genomes Project.* https://doi.org/10.17037/PUBS.04645534), the research and treasured exchanges with colleagues and peers thereafter helped me to refine and develop my thinking about what public trust in the health system is. The unconditional support of my family made this book possible. I would like to thank all who engaged with my work and hold this book in their hands.

I would like to thank Göran Tomson and Mesfin Kassaye Tessma from Karolinska Institute for their advice and support during the early years of my research. I thank my PhD supervisors Nicholas Mays and Sarah Smith, from the London School of Hygiene and Tropical Medicine, for their immensely valuable guidance throughout the years. I would like to thank Mary Dixon-Woods and Jenni Burt, from the University of Cambridge, who introduced me to the importance of signalling theory for trust building and for the opportunity to grow in academia. From the Swiss Federal Institute of Technology in Zurich, I would like to thank Effy Vayena, Alessandro Blasimme and the research team at the time, including Caroline Brall, Manuel Schneider, Marcello Ienca and Anna Jobin for the discussions about public trust in health data use and opportunities to mature my research portfolio. Thanks go to Viktor von Wyl, Markus Christen and the Digital Society Initiative community from the University of Zurich for the fruitful and highly supportive research environment that allows me to research public trust.

Thanks go to Heidi Larson from the London School of Hygiene and Tropical Medicine; Paola Daniore, Jana Sedlakova, Kimon Papadopoulos, Federica Zavattaro, Katrin Gille all from the University of Zurich; Georg Starke from the École polytechnique fédérale de Lausanne and Technical University of Munich; Vanja Pajić, independent expert in digital health in Zagreb; and Claudia Batz from the George Institute for Global Health for their valuable comments on different chapters of this book.

Appreciation goes to Laura Vickers-Rendall and Jay Allan, from Bristol University Press, for their guidance throughout the writing and publishing process of this book. I would like to thank the external reviewers of the book manuscript for their very helpful comments and guidance. Thanks also go to Georgina Asfaw for her copy editing during the publication process.

I thank the Digital Society Initiative, University of Zurich, for the DSI Postdoc Fellowship which allowed me to write this book.

ONE

Introduction

Trust is at the centre of the public and health system relationship. The public takes part in trusted health system activities and its trust legitimises health system activities. Examples of health system activities that particularly depend on high levels of public trust are data use in health care or public health interventions such as vaccination campaigns. Higher levels of public trust are associated with improved levels of population health, increased social cohesion, reduced system costs, well-functioning health system activities and a prosperous society. Lower levels of public trust can lead to decreasing levels of population health and risk health system failure. The main motivation for the public to trust the health system is the anticipation of a net benefit for the individual, society and the system. When considering the fundamental effects of public trust on the health system and the public's motivation to trust the health system, public trust should be considered as a central component during the health policy making process, when designing public health interventions and when acting as health professionals. In consideration of this, the aim of this book is to introduce and contextualise the main drivers of public trust in the health system.

Given the importance of public trust in health systems for both society and the system itself, the aim of describing public trust has motivated my research for several years. The basis of this book is built on the drive to provide an evidence-based description of the key components relevant for public trust in the health system. A conceptual understanding of public trust can help to a) inform health system activities, health policy making and health system governance; b) inform health communication; and c) inform public trust monitoring and evaluation. When I started to research public trust in the health system, there was limited understanding of what public trust is, despite the frequent use of the term in public media and debate. The use of the term 'public trust' in English language media suggested that public trust is a commonly understood concept, which was not the case. As one of my early incentives was to inform measurement scale development for public trust, my work has focused on improving conceptual precision in the field (MacKenzie, 2003; Wilson, 2005; Perron and Gillespie, 2015). Only if we have a rigorous understanding of public trust can we use the concept in a meaningful way to inform health system activities. If agreement is not found on a common understanding of public trust in health system activities, any further attempt to influence levels of public trust are close to meaningless.

Without doubt, at the time I started my research, a solid body of work described trust relationships in a variety of health care settings and countries, substantiated by research and trust theory from the political sciences, sociology, psychology and philosophy (O'Neill, 2002; Harrison, Innes and Zwanenberg, 2003; Hardin, 2006; Shore, 2006; Calnan and Rowe, 2008; Pilgrim, Tomasini and Vassilev, 2010). These works focused mainly on interpersonal trust relationships or the trust relationship of an individual and the system. Despite the available robust and eminent work on individual trust, I learned that the concept of public trust in the health system remained largely uncharted territory. The main difference between individual trust and public trust is that the former concept focuses on an individual's perspective towards the system or professional and the latter concept describes the relationship between 'the public' and 'the system'. Often, we find altruistic motivations and, as mentioned earlier, the anticipation of a net benefit as an outcome of the public–health system trust relationship. We need to acknowledge that scholars define trust differently and that a clear cut conceptual precision is hard to reach (Gille, Smith and Mays, 2014). For this book, I will regard public trust mostly as a separate concept from individual trust. Influenced by pioneering work on public trust in the German, Dutch, English and Welsh health system contexts by van der Schee and colleagues from 2007 (Schee et al, 2007; Schee, 2016), I started researching public trust by employing qualitative research methods and analysing trust theory in the context of the Swedish, English and Swiss health systems. To a large degree, the findings presented in this book are based on research conducted in the context of the English National Health Service (NHS). To conceptualise public trust, I analysed three qualitative case studies about data use in health care as part of my doctoral research at the London School of Hygiene and Tropical Medicine between 2013 and 2017, focusing on biobank research, genomics research and the failed introduction of care.data (Gille, 2017). The care.data programme was an NHS England initiative to provide better care to patients and support the UK research landscape. The programme failed to launch due to a range of concerns such as data safety and trustworthiness problems. Since 2017, I have researched trust and public trust in health system activities that depend on data use in the context of, for example, cross-border health data transfer, biobank research, genomics, health data cooperatives, digital research methods and artificial intelligence in medicine. At the time of the publication of this book, I research public trust in electronic health records in Austria, France, Germany, Italy, the Netherlands and Switzerland with a focus on European Public Health. All the insights from my previous and ongoing research on public trust in the health system find their way into this book.

To answer *What is Public Trust in the Health System?* the book is structured in three consecutive parts: Part I provides the background on the general concept of trust and should spark your interest in the topic of public trust. I consider part two as the core of the book. Part II builds on empirical and theoretical research on public trust in data use in health systems, where I present a full conceptual framework of public trust in the health system. Informed by the conceptual framework, Part III of the book proposes ways to build public trust in the health system through governance, communication and analysis. Following this Introduction chapter, Chapter Two answers the question *What are the basics of trust?* by explaining six basic components of trust. Chapter Three discusses contemporary case studies to showcase the role of public trust in the contexts of the COVID-19 pandemic, vaccination uptake and health data use in health system activities. The last case study, data use in health systems, will remain the focus of this book as an insightful health system activity to explain and discuss public trust in the health system. The chapters of Part II present a full conceptual framework of public trust in the health system. Chapter Four explains how public trust grows in the public sphere through open public discourse. Chapter Five describes what makes public trust. Chapter Six discusses legitimisation and acceptance as the outcomes of a trusting relationship between the public and the health system. The last chapter of Part II, Chapter Seven, illustrates issues that influence public trust building, but do not directly build public trust themselves. Anchored in the conceptual framework of public trust, Part III of this book suggests strategies to promote public trust in health system activities. Chapter Eight presents guiding principles for health system governance and policy making on how to foster public trust. As communication is the lifeblood of public trust, Chapter Nine, describes communication strategies that aim to promote public trust. Chapter Ten discusses ways to analyse public trust for health policy evaluation, performance analysis or quality improvement of care. Closing the book, the Conclusion chapter will summarise the main messages and points towards future research needs.

PART I

Why do we care about public trust in the health system?

Trust is significant for interhuman and intersocietal cooperation. The importance of trust extends to all areas of life and is not exclusive to the health system context. In February 1950, in Eleanor Roosevelt's television programme concerning the implications of the hydrogen bomb, Albert Einstein explained the fundamental role of trust for human cooperation: 'every kind of peaceful cooperation among men is primarily based on mutual trust and only secondarily on institutions such as courts of justice and police. This holds for nations as well as for individuals. And the basis of trust is loyal give and take' (Einstein, 1954, p 160). In the following two chapters I will discuss the basic components of trust to provide the background necessary to understand the more complex concept of public trust. Thereafter, I aim to show the importance of public trust with the help of three short health system related case studies.

TWO

What is trust?

To better understand what public trust is, I introduce the basic components of trust by examining trust-building among two parties. It is important to keep in mind that to this date no common agreement exists between scholars on how to define trust. In fact, the large quantity of literature on trust can be confusing (Taylor, Nong and Platt, 2023). This is not surprising as trust is context-specific, the composition of what builds trust is dynamic to adapt to ever changing environments, and our understanding of trust is formed by our upbringing, norms, values and culture. Consider for a moment for yourself, how do you describe trust in the context of your daily life?

We all have a personal understanding of what trust is, which makes the topic area initially easy to approach, but soon we will realise in discussions with others that it is not easy to come to a common understanding of trust. It is certainly possible that by the end of this chapter you agree with some points you read and question others. For example, when comparing a selection of established trust theories, we can read the following about trust:

> Trust functions so as to comprehend and reduce this complexity. (Luhmann, 2017, p 33)

Trust may be defined as confidence in the reliability of a person or system, regarding a given set of outcomes or events, where that confidence expresses a faith in the probity or love of another, or in the correctness of abstract principles (technical knowledge). (Giddens, 1990, p 34)

Trust is a bet about the future contingent actions of others. (Sztompka, 1999, p 25)

Trust is the expectation that arises within a community of regular, honest, and cooperative behaviour, based on commonly shared norms, on the part of other members of that community. Those norms can be about deep 'value' questions like the nature of God or justice, but they also encompass secular norms like professional standards and codes of behaviour. (Fukuyama, 1995, p 26)

To say we trust you means we believe you have the right intentions towards us and that you are competent to do what we trust you to do. (Hardin, 2006, p 17)

Scholars commonly conceptualise trust as a relational construct. To build trust we need past experiences, present perceptions and future anticipations towards a benefit. Trust usually relates to a degree of uncertainty as we do not know what the outcome of a trusting relationship will be. As a result, trust is inherently risky, and we are vulnerable towards betrayal of our trust by the trusted party. We also see that alternative constructs are used in trust theory and common language as if they are synonyms of trust (Abelson, Miller and Giacomini, 2009). Examples are 'I have faith in you', 'I have confidence in you' or 'I believe you can do it'. For reasons of simplification and conceptual clarity, I use the term trust only, often conjoined with words that provide an indication of the trust context, as in individual trust or public trust. To my understanding, faith describes faith in God in the religious context whereas trust in the context of religion refers to trust in the church as an institution or clerics as church representatives (Seligman, 1997). Confidence is a useful term to describe self-confidence, as a form of trust in our own capabilities and potential. Luhmann separated trust from confidence by explaining that in situations of choice, you trust, and in situations where you do not consider choices you have confidence in the overall system (Luhmann, 1988). The two concepts: self-confidence and general trust are both used in the health system context. On an individual level, self-confidence is important to be able to trust and to better cope with trust betrayal (Luhmann, 2017), and to exercise autonomy (Nys, 2015). Generalised trust allows us to engage better in spontaneous social interaction. The separation of belief and trust, or if one concept is part of the other concept, is a subject of philosophical debate (Hieronymi, 2008). It has also been examined how implicit beliefs of moral character can influence trust recovery, or how factual beliefs and trust in epistemic authorities influence each other (Haselhuhn, Schweitzer and Wood, 2010; Rekker and Harteveld, 2022). Acknowledging the ongoing research and debates about belief and trust, I suggest separating the concepts and not using both interchangeably. A last observation we can make is that modern trust theories move within a two-by-two matrix, describing an individual and public focus of trust, as well as the decision to place trust motivated either by emotions or calculated decisions. A deeper semantic and historic analysis of the word trust and similar terms is interesting, but beyond the scope of this book (Frevert, 2013).

Drawing from existing work, I argue that six components make up the basic components of trust relationships, as presented in order of the trust establishment process in Table 2.1 (Gille, 2022).

Knowing about such trust components helps to navigate trust conceptualisations in several ways. First, we increase the understandability of complex trust conceptualisations by being able to identify the basic trust components. Second,

Table 2.1: Universal trust components

Universal trust components	*Explanations*
Relationship	*We need a relation to trust*
Communication	*We need to communicate to place trust*
Truth	*We need truthful information to place trust*
Autonomy	*We need free choice to place trust*
Alternatives	*We need alternatives between which we choose to trust*
No guarantee	*We cannot guarantee trust*

Source: Adapted from Gille 2022

being familiar with the core components of trust will help us to develop more complex and abstract conceptual frameworks of trust as we can easily identify the basic starting point. Third, when comparing a range of conceptual frameworks of trust in a similar health care context, we can better identify what is common and what is different between such conceptualisations. Fourth, linked to the previous point, we will be able to better transfer conceptualisations between different contexts when we know about the commonalities and differences of trust conceptualisations. When considering the context specificity and dynamic characteristics of trust, I suggest it is worthwhile to keep a reflexive and open mindset while researching trust (Möllering, 2001). A narrow and rigid understanding of trust will stall research and policy processes. This is because when comparing or transferring trust conceptualisations between settings we will seldomly experience a perfect fit and therefore are required to adapt, validate or develop new trust conceptualisations for new settings.

Relationship – *we need a relation to trust*

We place trust in someone or something. If there is no other to place trust in, trust cannot be established. In its most simple form, a trust relationship is: A trusts B to do or not to do X (Hardin, 1993, 1999). For example, A is a patient (the trusting party) in need of a positive outcome that she cannot reach by her own means and skills; B is the physician (trusted party) with the necessary skills to reach the positive outcome for the patient; and X is the patient's anticipated positive outcome of a medical procedure performed by the physician. This linear understanding of a trust relationship can be expanded in situations of reciprocal trust where B also trusts A to reach a common benefit X. Examples are a physician trusting the patient's information to inform a treatment decision (Groenewegen, Hansen and Jong, 2019); or a doctor trusting a patient's competence (Thorne and Robinson, 1988). Building this trust relationship model a little further, we see the introduction of a trust focus either in terms of a specific task we trust someone with, or a specific circumstance we trust someone in (Starke et al, 2022). Therefore, we usually do not issue trust as a general free-ride ticket for the trusted party, but we place trust in the trusted party to perform a specific task. Similarly, we place trust in specific circumstances of need, but when such circumstances change, we might not need to trust any more. This differentiation allows us to trust a person in some areas and simultaneously not to trust the same person in other areas. For example, I trust my five-year-old son to walk to the bakery around the corner to buy bread, but I do not trust my son to cycle downtown to go grocery shopping. When the circumstances change and he competently navigates his bike in traffic, I will trust him to cycle downtown to go grocery shopping.

This simple two-party model of a trust relationship being built at the individual level helps us to understand the basics of trust. In the context of health care and health systems, such trust relationships are most of the time complex, involve multiple actors and are dynamic (Meyer et al, 2008). The relational complexity develops from the complexity of the health system or health care activities themselves where several actors are involved in the health care process. Furthermore, we see that trust not only develops among two parties in a linear relationship, but often third parties, and knowledge about regulations or governance structures, come into play as system guarantees. When we refer to individual trust in a hospital or system, such trust can be established via personal relationships between individuals and hospital staff who are considered as hospital and/or system representatives. Also, trust can be established by knowledge about existing quality criteria, professional codes, oversight processes or hospital accreditation processes, all of which might be understood as guarantees for trustworthiness. It is likely we build trust by both personal relationships and system guarantees (Kroeger, 2017; Topp et al, 2022). In the context of Zambian primary health centres, we see that providers' workplace trust develops from a complex interplay of trust in employer, trust in supervisor and trust in colleagues. In the same context, patient–provider trust is influenced not only by interpersonal trust between patients and providers but also by institutional trust (Topp and Chipukuma, 2016). In the emerging research area of user trust in artificial intelligence applications in medicine, as for example when used in clinical imaging in dermatology, clinical neuroscience or in artificial intelligence-supported health chatbots, we see that conceptual clarity is still missing to a large degree (Gille, Jobin and Ienca, 2020; Starke, 2021; Sedlakova and Trachsel, 2022). While some argue that trust is an interhuman concept and therefore trust in artificial intelligence is conceptual nonsense, human-computer action research suggests that the concept of user trust in artificial intelligence is worth elaborating further (Starke et al, 2022). Empirical and theoretical conceptual research in that field has just started to emerge, arguing both in favour of and against the use of the concept of trust in artificial intelligence, as well as covering ideas of direct trust relationships and multi-actor relationships, or approaching the debate by analyses of distrust and misplaced trust (Ferrario, Loi and Viganò, 2020; Ryan,

2020; Starke and Ienca, 2022). These examples show on the one hand that trust in the context of health systems usually develops in a complex interaction network, and on the other hand that trust conceptualisations in some areas of health system activities are in their early development stages, which reminds us to be careful when making assumptions about trust relationships in different health care settings.

We can conclude that trust is a relational construct that requires at least one other party in which we place trust. In the health system context, trust typically develops in a network of relationships.

Communication – *we need to communicate to place trust*

Communication is the lifeblood of trust relationships. Without exchanging information, trust cannot be established, as indicated by many conceptualisations of trust that incorporate communication and our own experience (Mechanic, 1996; Pearson and Raeke, 2000; Ozawa and Sripad, 2013). By the means of communication, we obtain the information about the to be trusted that is necessary to place trust. In interpersonal relationships, communication helps us to get to know each other and to develop expectations towards each other. Within societies, communication will help us to build a consensus which is important for the development of public trust (Gilson, 2006). Communication takes place in various formats, by a) exchanging words, b) recognising signals and signs, and c) processing personal and collective experiences in our memories during the trust-building process. We exchange words during conversations with health care professionals or acquire information by reading or listening to news in the public or social media (Schee, Jong and Groenewegen, 2012; Pérez-Escoda et al, 2020). Similarly, we gain information about others' trustworthiness by intentionally displayed signals and subtle signs (Bacharach and Gambetta, 2001; Gambetta, 2011). The display of a well-known and reputable label can build trust, as can neat work clothing. Signs that communicate trust-building features, such as skill, integrity or predictability, foster trust in emergent relationships (Branzei, Vertinsky and Camp, 2007). What should not be neglected is the third information source that is our own and our collective memory. Prior experiences exchanged during discussions with others or pulled back from our memory during our own reflection are a key driver for trust (Gilson, Palmer and Schneider, 2005; Mattila and Rapeli, 2018). As one example of collective memories shows, present African American perspectives on breast cancer and its treatment are among other factors influenced by collective memories of past medical experimentations and their harmful impact on the African American community. 'The social barriers to perceived access, then, entail fears and distrust of health care providers based on personal and community-based experience and collective memory of poor, unfair treatment' (Ferrera et al, 2016, p 462).

In summary, we use different means of communication to gather information to build trust: we talk, listen and read; we use information provided by signs and signals; and we process our own and others' past comparable experiences.

Truth – *we need truthful information to place trust*

The purpose of trust-building communication is to convey truthful information. Such information covers a range of different themes that develop from the underlying trust concept in the given setting. This can be about public trust in health information sharing (Platt, Jacobson and Kardia, 2018), patients' trust in primary care providers (Hall et al, 2002), trust in micro-health insurance (Schneider, 2005), trust in medical artificial intelligence (Starke et al, 2022), public trust in the health system (Gille, Smith and Mays, 2020), and so on. For example, a systematic review of 45 trust in the health system measures showed that the most dominant themes of trust in the health system are quality and nature of *communication*;

level of integrity and openness perceived as *honesty*; *confidence* developing from a belief in reliability; *competence*; *fidelity*; *system trust* developing from a belief in institutions' processes and policies; *confidentiality* maintained by privacy; and treatment *fairness* (Ozawa and Sripad, 2013, p 12). At the same time, such information needs to be perceived as truthful by the trusting party to assess the trustworthiness of the other.

Such a dominant focus on communication of truth has caveats. How can we assess truthful information? How do we deal with conflicting professional advice which we consider as truthful in both instances? How do we know that we are not dealing with a swindler? How do we deal with the problem that different people judge truth differently leading to problems associated with multiple truth? How do we deal with conspiracy theories and fake news competing against truthful information in the public space (Waszak, Kasprzycka-Waszak and Kubanek, 2018)? What if professionals perceive truth telling as an ethical dilemma (Zhang and Min, 2020)? Those questions show the difficulty of truth telling and truth assessment. From a receiver point of view, we will not be able to assess if we are told the truth to an absolute certainty. Consequently, placing trust can be a gamble. To increase certainty about the truthfulness of information, we have several processes implemented in health systems as well as control mechanisms at our own disposal. Telling the truth is a basic moral rule in health systems and therefore deeply rooted in professional ethics, yet cultural differences and balancing what is best for a patient can influence truth-telling behaviour (Pergert and Lützén, 2012). We have started to teach college students methods on how to identify fake news and we can access fact-checking webpages to identify if facts in the public sphere are true or not (Musgrove et al, 2018). Ongoing discussions about the role of social media platforms for deliberative democracies raise public awareness about the risks of fake news. The purpose shift of such platforms from communication platforms for private customers to public forums for democratic citizenship has initiated reconsiderations among platform designers and owners (Chambers, 2021). We know that health literacy on the receiver end, and accessible communication by the sender, are critical to truth (Netemeyer et al, 2020).

Truthful information about what makes someone or something trustworthy is imperative to trust establishment. Simultaneously, assessing the truth and telling the truth is not always easy. Therefore, trust remains a risky choice.

Autonomy – *we need free choice to place trust*

Trust grows in free relationships and from free will (Misztal, 1996). Autonomy to choose is an integral concept of medical ethics, as demonstrated by the informed consent process. In fact, some understand that the signature on a consent form is a sign of trust (O'Neill, 2002). In situations in which we place trust, it is always upon others to assess whether someone is trustworthy (Hartmann, 1994). An expectation to be trusted or forcing someone into trust is illogical and will not lead to trust. Yet, situations exist where we cannot exercise our autonomy. For example, if we are unconscious, we have no alternatives to choose from or we do not have the time to choose, as for example in emergency care situations (Meyer and Ward, 2013). In such situations, trust is replaced by other concepts such as dependence (discussed in the next section) or confidence in the system, or trust is mediated by others such as trusted family members that act in the interest of the unconscious patient. Further, ethical guidelines and professional conduct come into use as system guarantees of professionals' trustworthy behaviour.

Alternatives – *we need alternatives between which we choose to trust*

We need alternatives to make choices. We trust one physician over other physicians. For Luhmann, the ability to make choices when placing trust is imperative (Luhmann, 1988, 2009). A qualitative study on patient trust in public and private hospitals in South Australia shows that choice and trust are tied together for private patients. However, for patients in the public part of the health system that cannot make choices, the researchers described that trust emerges as a form of 'resigned trust' due to a lack of alternatives and dependence on the health system (Ward et al, 2015). Some of the same authors found in an earlier study that in many situations there is simply no choice in the health system and patients depend on the system. They concluded that dependence is not a 'negative construct but rather, similar to trust, dependence may be understood as a means of coping with uncertainty by reducing complexity' (Meyer and Ward, 2013, p 291). We also see choice experiments being used in a range of research studies on trust and underlying trust concepts, especially in behavioural economics and psychology, placing choice at the centre of trust research.

No guarantee – *we cannot guarantee trust*

We can do a lot of things right and act to the best of our knowledge to be a trustworthy partner, but there will never be a guarantee that someone trusts us. Mainly this is because we are not assessing our own trustworthiness (Hartmann, 1994). It is always upon others to place trust in us. Furthermore, trust is not always the only reason why people engage in a relationship or interact with something. Consider, for example, a range of equally trustworthy services, but people choose a service that is conveniently located close to their home. We might use an online communication application, despite privacy concerns, because we want to be part of a group and not lose contact with others who use the application. Usually, other concepts beside trust exist that can lead to acceptance, relationship-building or use of services. To my knowledge, no study exists that shows a guaranteed way of how to establish trust. This awareness is helpful to adjust expectations when implementing guidelines that aim to increase trustworthiness, such as some ethics guidelines for artificial intelligence (Jobin, Ienca and Vayena, 2019). For years we have observed the push towards more transparency, as for example in biobank research (Gille, Axler and Blasimme, 2020) or governments more broadly (O'Neill, 2003; Boufides, Gable and Jacobson, 2019). Did such mechanisms always lead to higher levels of trust? Depending on the context, we can observe the formation of public and professional perceptions of low levels of trust or even the emergence of a trust crisis in health care (Shore, 2006; van der Meer, 2017).

Trust remains a vital construct for relationship building and social cohesion, yet there is no guarantee that trust is established despite our best actions and knowledge on how to be trustworthy.

Concluding remarks

This chapter discussed basic components of trust to set the stage for further explorations of trust in a range of different contexts. Trust is a complex, dynamic and context-specific construct that is shaped by our own life experiences, as well as the norms and values of the society we live in. I proposed that basic components of trust are relationship building, communication of truthful information, making autonomous choices among alternatives, and that trust cannot be guaranteed. I consider truthful information about what makes someone or something trustworthy of utmost importance for the trust-building process. At the same time, making a free choice to place trust is central to trust-building processes.

THREE

Three health system examples: vaccination uptake, COVID-19 pandemic and health data use in health systems

Public trust in the health system describes a relational construct in which we anticipate that a trusted health care activity will have a positive effect on ourselves and others. We participate in trusted health care actions and thereby contribute, with our own actions, towards the improvement of the population's health. Vaccination programmes, non-pharmaceutical interventions to fight the COVID-19 pandemic and health data use in the health system are health system activities which are particularly suitable to show the importance of public trust. Health system actions have not only a personal effect but also a public effect in the three case studies. Public interest, altruistic motivations and net-benefits are common, but not exclusive, characteristics of health care activities that depend on public trust.

Public trust in vaccination

Vaccination is one of the most important health system activities to promote population health. Ample scientific research supports vaccinations' effectiveness, efficacy and safety (Deml et al, 2019). On a global scale, vaccination eradicates diseases and drastically reduces global mortality. For example, according to the World Health Organisation (WHO), vaccination against measles alone prevented 23 million deaths between 2010 and 2018 (World Health Organization, 2020). Despite the abundant evidence that vaccinations are highly effective as protective intervention against vaccine-preventable diseases, in 2019, the WHO named vaccine hesitancy as one of the top ten threats to global health (World Health Organization, 2019), given the risks of low levels of vaccination coverage for outbreaks of vaccine-preventable diseases (de Figueiredo et al, 2020). According to a 2016 international comparative survey study in 67 countries, confidence in vaccines differs across the globe. Survey respondents in France were the least confident about vaccine safety, while Bangladesh had the highest confidence in vaccine safety. Results from Bangladesh, Ecuador and Iran showed the highest reported agreement about vaccination being important for disease prevention, whereas respondents in Azerbaijan, Russia and Italy had a lower reported agreement about vaccine importance (Larson et al, 2016, p 297).

Dating back to the mid-1800s, vaccine hesitancy has walked hand in hand with the development and administration of vaccines (Larson et al, 2011). Vaccine hesitancy, although no commonly agreed definition exists, can be understood as:

> a behaviour, influenced by a number of factors including issues of confidence (level of trust in vaccine or provider), complacency (do not perceive a need for a vaccine, do not value the vaccine), and convenience (access). Vaccine-hesitant individuals are a heterogeneous group that are indecisive in varying degrees about specific vaccines or

vaccination in general. (European Centre for Disease Prevention and Control, 2017, p 1)

As the quote describes, vaccine hesitancy is a multifaceted problem that is challenging to describe and to address. Models describing vaccine hesitancy portray trust as a dominant factor influencing the degree of vaccine hesitancy (World Health Organization Strategic Advisory Group of Experts (SAGE) on Immunization, 2014). In the current WHO Immunization Agenda 2030, public trust and confidence remain a key focus area (World Health Organization, 2020).

Vijayaprasad Gopichandran identified six possible factors that may lead to mistrust in vaccination in the Indian context in 2017: 1) increasing scepticism towards science and technology, which develops from the difficulty to separate beliefs and facts, an increasing 'post-truth' environment in politics and suspicion about evidence generation; 2) availability of strong alternative schools of thought, which focus on passing on beliefs in the power of natural remedies and avoidance of chemical substances such as vaccines; 3) misinformation regarding vaccination, which can spread faster than truthful information; 4) influence of the internet and social media, where adverse events and misinformation spread across the country; 5) perception of conflicts of interest in vaccine policy, such as potential ties between the pharma industry, vaccination policy makers and professional bodies; and 6) perceived lack of transparency and openness about adverse vaccination events during vaccine trials (Gopichandran, 2017, pp 101–2). The six factors are transferable to other societies outside of India and provide a good overview of the complex societal factors that can lead to mistrust in vaccination. The causes leading to mistrust in vaccination are rooted in a range of socio-political activities far outside of the health system context. Heidi Larson and colleagues state that 'the interconnectivity of vaccine confidence, confidence in the health system, public trust in government more broadly, and socio-economic status alongside the influences of religious and philosophical beliefs, suggest that measuring vaccine confidence can be a valuable window on bigger issues at play in the evolving health and development landscape' (Larson et al, 2016, p 300).

What is public trust in vaccination?

In 2018, Larson and colleagues described public trust in vaccination as a construct that emerges from a triangular relationship of trust in the vaccination product, vaccination provider and policy maker (as health system representative). Historic trust, generalised trust and external influencers have an effect on this trust triangle. Firstly, historic trust emerges from the collective memory of discrimination against, for example, several minority groups over a sustained time period. Secondly, generalised trust describes the ability of individuals to trust others in society and is often associated with social capital. Lastly, external influencers which are non-official sources, such as family members or public figures, can also influence trust (Larson et al, 2018). In 2016, and featuring similar factors, Sachiko Ozawa and colleagues developed a complex model to describe the role of trust and communication on the utilisation of vaccines and the health system (Ozawa, Paina and Qiu, 2016). Their model builds on: 'trust in vaccination, trust in health systems, health and immunization system readiness, positive and negative communication arising from community sources and more broadly from sources outside the community (i.e. media, government), and utilization of both vaccines and the health system' (Ozawa, Paina and Qiu, 2016, p 133). Both conceptualisations of public trust in vaccination show how a complex network of actors and diverse trust relationships within and between societies form perceptions of trust.

What builds trust in vaccination?

No silver bullet exists to build public trust where it is lost. This applies especially to public trust in vaccines, which navigates a complex network of relationships and actors. Across the literature we find a broad set of strategies to address misinformation and conspiracy about vaccination programs. For example, the WHO suggests that stakeholder engagement and communication between health professionals and patients can act as a mechanism to build trust in vaccinations (World Health Organization, 2017a). Similarly, a recent study that investigated different mechanisms to increase COVID-19 vaccination rates among unvaccinated American Christians found that health professionals mentioning a common religious identity to their patients motivates religious patient groups to place higher trust in the medical professional, as well as to have a greater intention to get vaccinated and promote vaccinations among friends and family (Chu, Pink and Willer, 2021). In Japan, which has one of the lowest levels of confidence in the human papillomavirus (HPV) vaccine, a 2021 study recommended a multi-stakeholder approach to overcome the HPV vaccine hesitancy. This strategy involved incorporating the national and local government, professional organisations, politicians, civil society and mass media. The actors' involvement focused on communication, shared narratives, engagement and education (Kunitoki et al, 2021).

Strategies to overcome vaccine hesitancy and to build public trust in vaccination aim at building cohesion among vaccine hesitant citizens and professional groups. Potentially helpful mechanisms to support the trust building include communication of information and shared narratives, engaging different stakeholders in decision-making processes, educating the public and showing shared identity cues.

Public trust in non-pharmaceutical interventions to fight the COVID-19 pandemic

'Globally, as of 12:14pm CEST, 12 July 2023, there have been 767,972,961 confirmed cases of COVID-19, including 6,950,655 deaths, reported to WHO. As of 9 July 2023, a total of 13,462,024,421 vaccine doses have been administered' (World Health Organization, 2023). The United Nations emphasised that the COVID-19 pandemic is the biggest challenge for global society since World War II (United Nations, 2020). In response to the pandemic, governments across the globe introduced non-pharmaceutical interventions to control the growing numbers of COVID-19 positive cases and to slow down the spread of airborne virus transmissions (Greenhalgh et al, 2021; Liu et al, 2022). Non-pharmaceutical interventions were necessary to control viral spread before vaccines started to become available in late 2020 and the beginning of 2021. Following different approaches in the early phases of the pandemic, the interventions harmonised across most countries over time. The interventions included movement interventions, such as national travel restrictions; physical and social distancing interventions, such as cancellation of church services; personal protective interventions, such as face masks; and special protection interventions to shield vulnerable risk groups (Sabat et al, 2020; Wang and Mao, 2021). The wide range of interventions introduced enormous pressures on societies, affecting mental health and causing ethical, economic, social and political challenges. The interventions especially targeted vulnerable populations to protect them against COVID-19 (Bellazzi and Boyneburgk, 2020; Sekalala et al, 2020).

Studies show that, aside from perceived risks, public trust in governments and science communities is a key contributor to public acceptance and adoption of COVID-19 interventions (Cairney and Wellstead, 2020; Dohle, Wingen and Schreiber, 2020; Plohl and Musil, 2020; Devine et al, 2021; Pagliaro et al, 2021; Siegrist and Bearth, 2021; Hensel et al, 2022). The history of epidemics also taught us that public trust is critical for a successful fight to end epidemics, and that epidemics can also be used as opportunities to build trust between the science community and society (Celum et al, 2020). Trust in the government and health system is a critical factor in fighting the Ebola virus (Farrar and Piot, 2014; Blair, Morse and Tsai, 2017), the severe acute respiratory syndrome (SARS) outbreak in the early 2000s (Deurenberg-Yap et al, 2005; Lee, 2009), the human immunodeficiency viruses (HIV) (Whetten et al, 2008), and the influenza A virus subtype H1N1 (van der Weerd et al, 2011).

What is public trust in non-pharmaceutical interventions to fight the COVID-19 pandemic?

Building on Earle and colleagues' Trust-Confidence-Cooperation model that describes risk management in organisations, Gopichandran and colleagues suggest that cooperation with public health interventions in the Indian context during the COVID-19 pandemic is influenced by an interplay of trust and confidence in the health system. Shared values and the belief that the health system will protect the community and acts in the public's best interest builds trust. It builds upon past positive experiences with the health system (Earle and Siegrist, 2008; Earle, 2010; Gopichandran, Subramaniam and Kalsingh, 2020). Studies confirm the importance of past experiences and general levels of trust in the health system prior to a pandemic. Both have an impact on trust levels in the health system and pandemic management during the pandemic (Apeti, 2022; Makowska, Boguszewski and Podkowińska, 2022). However, according to a global study, 'trust in science can promote people's policy approval of new rules, but has only a small, indirect effect on adherence to these rules' (Sulik et al, 2021, p 8).

The combination of positive experiences with the health system and the anticipation of positive outcomes resulting from government actions in the public interest are common factors to public trust-building in health systems. Aspects that are not covered in Gopichandran and colleagues' model are appropriate risk communication and community co-development of interventions to build trust in such interventions (World

Health Organization, 2022c). As many pandemic interventions have a fundamental impact on the livelihood of different communities, such interventions need to be practical to be acceptable. Interventions that do not work in practice, as well as interventions that are not explained appropriately to the public, or that appear arbitrary, undermine public trust in the government. In comparison to public trust in vaccination programmes, public trust in non-pharmaceutical interventions is likely less dependent on personal relationships with medical professionals. Whereas medical professionals certainly can have an impact on trust in such interventions, especially when patients ask them about their opinion or when medical professionals and scientists appear on public media, the implementation of non-pharmaceutical interventions does not directly depend on health system professionals as the administration of a vaccine does.

What builds public trust in non-pharmaceutical interventions to fight the COVID-19 pandemic?

As mistrust leads to lower acceptance of pandemic interventions, which has adverse health effects on populations, Gopichandran and colleagues argue that 'public trust in the health system during pandemic times becomes an ethical imperative' (Gopichandran, Subramaniam and Kalsingh, 2020, p 214). Suggested actions to build public trust in pandemic interventions include risk communication related to the pandemic interventions, community engagement and health system activities in the public interest. Such actions produce positive outcomes that lead to positive public experiences of the management of the ongoing pandemic. The knowledge of trusted public health providers being involved in the development of COVID-19 contact tracing apps built public trust in the UK (Horvath, Banducci and James, 2022). Last, and not in our hands anymore, are previous positive experiences with the health system. Public trust cannot be stockpiled on a shelf for future public health emergencies, but knowledge of the importance of past positive experiences makes a strong case to continuously take public trust building seriously in preparedness of future intervention.

Public trust in health data use in health systems

The digital transformation and introduction of digital health in health systems is quickly expanding (Kickbusch, 2019). Referring to the US Food and Drug Administration, Adjekum and colleagues describe digital health as 'comprising of mHealth, wearable devices, telehealth, telemedicine, personalized medicine, electronic health records (EHRs), and health information technology' (Adjekum, Blasimme and Vayena, 2018, p 2). With the introduction of digital health in health systems, many anticipate various benefits but also risks for the individual, society and system (World Health Organization, 2021). Commonly anticipated benefits are improved quality, safety and access to health care, reduced health care costs or the improved ability to personalise health care. In contrast, digital health also results in emerging digitalisation gaps, which may lead to inequity and access barriers, foremost in relation to age, gender, ethnicity, disability, socioeconomic status or geographical location (OECD, 2018; Elena-Bucea et al, 2021; van Kessel et al, 2022).

Common to the wide range of current digital health interventions is the pivotal importance to collect, aggregate, store and process data from both healthy and ill citizens (Vayena et al, 2018). What counts as data is an ever-evolving category of structured and unstructured data comprising of, for example, data about medication, diagnoses, medical procedures, genetics, social history, lifestyle or the environment (Weber, Mandl and Kohane, 2014). When we implement digital health innovations such as EHRs, one of the backbones of digital health, we are confronted with not only regulatory and technological challenges, but also with societal and ethical challenges. Influenced by the public perception of these challenges, public trust is at the forefront and a core issue for the successful implementation and use of data-driven health system activities (Gasser et al, 2020; Ghafur et al, 2020; Foley et al, 2021; Belfrage, Helgesson and Lynøe, 2022). If such activities suffer from insufficient levels of public trust, these activities are at the risk of failing because of people not participating in such activities.

What is public trust in health data use in health systems?

Public trust in health data use can be understood as:

> a concept that grows in the public sphere from open public discourse and, as a result, legitimises the actions of health systems. Public trust builds on information equally relating to past experiences, present perceptions and future expectations. Public trust is established in anticipation of a net-benefit for the public as well as the system. (Gille and Brall, 2020, p 233; Gille, Smith and Mays, 2020)

Underlying this definition is a full conceptual framework of public trust in the health system presented in Part II of this book. As the definition shows, public trust is a public discourse-based construct. In the context of public trust building to enable the use of digital proximity tracing apps in Singapore, Gordon Kuo Siong Tan and Sun Sun Lim emphasise the significance of dialogic communication in its capacity to build relationships (Tan and Lim, 2022). In the public sphere, which typically entails online and physical communication fora, it is common practice to engage with members of the public and actors from within and outside the health system to discuss trust issues of mutual interest. Examples of engagement methods are citizen juries or public deliberation events where health system actors and citizens come together (Geisler, 2022). Nancy Baum and colleagues explained in 2009 how public deliberation methods in south-east Michigan, US, helped to build public trust in social distancing measures during a pandemic (Baum, Jacobson and Goold, 2009). Public deliberation methods are most useful when policy is characterised by 'conflicting public values, high controversy, combined expert and real-world knowledge, and low trust in government' (Solomon and Abelson, 2012, p 1). By building on health system experiences, the present understanding of the health system's potential to fulfil the trusted action, and the anticipation of a benefit for the trusters (the individual, the system and the society), it is possible to arrive at a collective understanding of trust. Jodyn Platt and Sharon Kardia proposed a model of public trust in health information sharing which identifies the following trust-building mechanisms as characteristics of those placing trust: a) knowledge of information sharing; b) experience with the health system; c) privacy concerns; d) expectations of benefits; e) propensity to trust; f) demographics. All characteristics influence health system trust in combination with fidelity, integrity, competence and global trust (Platt and Kardia, 2015, fig 1). The model is helpful to understand the distinctive characteristics of trust building in data dependent activities as compared to other activities. Specifically, trust in data dependent activities can be enabled through a reasonable comprehension of the data information sharing activity and privacy protection mechanisms.

What builds public trust in health data use in health systems?

Guided by conceptual definitions that describe key enablers of public trust in a digital health activity, we can implement a range of mechanisms that can contribute to trustworthiness in the use of health data in health systems. Such mechanisms usually cover topics of data security and privacy protection, offering autonomy to the user to make decisions about data use, explanatory transparency about data use processes, and providing information about expected benefits of the data use. The precise set of public trust-building mechanisms depends on the context, and there is no generic blueprint. However, in my research and in Chapter Eight of this book I suggest that a range of higher order guiding principles for health system actors are helpful for the trust-building process, which are (Gille, Smith and Mays, 2022): 1) Do not rush trust building, as it requires time to build trust. It is impossible to enforce public trust or demand public trust; 2) Engage with the public to communicate information and build relationships. Building public trust needs more than just being trustworthy, it requires relationship building between the public and health system representatives (Samuel et al, 2021); 3) Keep the public safe and protect their data; 4) Offer autonomy to the public so that people can decide if they want to take part in digital health activities or not; 5) Plan for diverse trust relationships, as the public trusts different health system actors to a different degree. For example, politicians are generally less trusted than frontline medical staff. Yet both can play a role in trust building in health data activities. Therefore, a holistic approach is necessary that factors in such differences and tailors trust-building mechanisms to the different actors; 6) Recognise that trust is shaped by both emotional and rational thought. Most public trust research portrays public trust as a construct that develops from calculative thinking. Next to this research, a body of literature describes trust building as an emotional process. Both processes require carefully tailored but aligned mechanisms and activities to reach a common output to enable public trust; 7) Represent the public interest and work with a public benefit-oriented mindset; and 8) Work towards realising a net-benefit for the health system and the public. It is important for the public to understand what the expected benefit will be to build trust. Otherwise, why should the public trust the use of their data in health systems if there is no clear benefit?

Concluding remarks

All three real life examples in this chapter show the importance of public trust for the success of health system activities. There is no one-size-fits-all approach to public trust building due to the context specificity of the construct. Fortunately, we can distil a range of overarching public trust-building mechanisms and principles from research findings. Public trust develops not only from being a trustworthy health system but also from engagement between health system actors and the public. Reccurring topics in the trust-building process are positive experiences, communication, weighing up risks, safety and privacy, public interest, benevolence and anticipated future benefits.

By drilling deeper into the field of public trust in data use in health systems, the following chapters will discuss in detail what public trust in the health system is and what mechanisms can build public trust in the health system.

PART II

What is public trust in the health system?

Where does public trust develop and what is public trust? Two crucial questions to answer when we want to understand the public trust concept. Conceptual precision is needed as 'a clear definition of the concept of trust is necessary in order to measure it' (OECD, 2017, p 35). The same is true for policy making, to design communication strategies and simply to talk about public trust. There is little value in aiming to work on public trust when we do not know what public trust is. We can observe in recent years a rise in the occurrence of the term trust in public debate. Despite the importance of the concept for health system performance, as well as the public wish to discuss issues of trust, we see that trust is oftentimes almost used as an eye-catching buzzword. Trust appears in marketing across all areas of life, and this inflationary use of the term trust can diminish its value. When we talk about trust and public trust, we should be considerate and only use trust where appropriate (Gille and Brall, 2020). On many occasions we might initially think that trust is the right concept in focus. Yet, maybe there are other better-fitting concepts that are closely linked to trust, but different, such as reliance, expectation, or dependence; see Chapter Two. A good understanding of public trust can help in public debates to draw the conceptual boundaries of public trust, as well as to identify if trust is used as a buzzword or in meaningful debate.

Chapter Four will explain how public trust develops in the public sphere and Chapters Five, Six and Seven will present a full conceptual framework of public trust in the health system. The conceptual framework builds largely on the research conducted for my doctoral thesis. I synthesised the conceptual framework from the results of an inductive analysis of three qualitative case studies about personal data use in the English NHS, as well as trust theory developed in the social and political sciences (Elo and Kyngäs, 2008; Gille, 2017). Throughout this process, priority was given to the data emerging from the following case studies: in the first case study, I analysed 1,625 readership comments relating to 58 online news articles (BBC n = 2; Daily Mail n = 16; Guardian n = 14; Independent n = 15; Telegraph n = 11) collected in 2015 about the NHS England care.data programme; in the second case study, I conducted a secondary analysis of 21 participant interviews run in 2011 about experiences and perceptions of contributing to biobank research (Locock and Boylan, 2016); in the third case study, I analysed data from two public focus groups[1] about perceptions of the 100,000 Genomes Project (Ryan et al, 2020). Public trust is important for all three health system activities to work. Care.data was an attempt by NHS England to introduce a patient data sharing infrastructure between 2013 and 2016. Care.data had several objectives, for example to improve quality of care and enable research. Due to several controversies and concerns raised about project objectives, opt-out consent, public communication, data use, planning and security, the project was abandoned (Hays and Daker-White, 2015; National Data Guardian, 2016). Issues of care.data trustworthiness were reccurring topics in public debate. Biobanks, which are repositories of biological samples and donor data, depend on the willingness of the public to donate their data for research (Shaw, Elger and Colledge, 2014). Public trust is understood to be a critical component of the biobanks' success (Tutton, Kaye and Hoeyer, 2004; Hawkins and O'Doherty, 2010). The 100,000 Genomes Project, run by Genomics England, aims to develop genomic medicine to transform delivery of care (Genomics England, 2022). As the name indicates, 'the principal objective of the 100,000 Genomes Project was to sequence 100,000 genomes from patients with cancers, rare disorders, and infectious disease, and to link the sequence data to a standardised, extensible account of diagnosis, treatment and outcomes' (Ryan et al, 2020, p 6). Like biobank research, the 100,000 Genomes Project also depends on donor and public trust (Samuel and Farsides, 2018a, 2018b).

The full conceptual framework comprises of three parts: a) causal themes that describe what builds public trust; b) effect themes that describe the outcome of a trusting public and health system relationship; and c) framing themes that describe what influences public trust building (Figure II.1).

It is important to include all themes of the three categories when working with the concept and not to use a subset of themes unless justified by the context the concept is applied to. Application of the concept to other health system activities

Figure II.1: Visualisation of how causal, effect and framing themes relate to each other

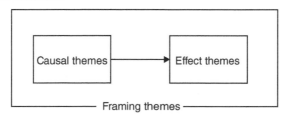

Source: Adapted from Gille, Smith and Mays 2020

outside of health data use or entire health systems is certainly possible and desirable, but such transfer processes require careful adaptation following established methods (Harachi et al, 2006; Sidani et al, 2010). The underlying data of the conceptual framework presented in this book originated from the United Kingdom and my recent research experience suggests that the conceptual framework works in countries with similar norms and values as well as similar understandings of what a health system is. As one example, preliminary and unpublished findings of my ongoing research project on public trust in electronic health records in Switzerland and other European countries suggests that the concept is robust, useful for the context of electronic health records and works well in neighbouring countries of Switzerland. I am therefore optimistic that the following chapters will be informative for a range of health system settings, and a wide spectrum of data driven health system activities other than the case studies the data emerged from.

Note

[1]   The focus group data used for this research was collected as part of a research project funded by the Department of Health (DH), through its funding of the Policy Innovation Research Unit at the London School of Hygiene and Tropical Medicine. All views expressed are those of the author and are not necessarily those of the DH.

FOUR

Where does public trust develop?

Trust between two individuals most of the time develops during conversations with each other, over shared positive experiences, or through shared personal characteristics such as identity, upbringing, education, culture, norms and values. We may work together with colleagues to reach a common goal and, over time, during this work process we get to know each other well, coming to conclusions about each other's trustworthiness which leads to a trust relationship. This process can be implicit and not necessarily something we think about much, but we might also come to a somewhat calculated decision to place trust. During the decision process we weigh possible risks of betrayal against an expected optimal benefit. We experience this trust building in our families, among friends, in our professional and social life. According to Erik Erikson's stages of psychosocial development, we learn what trust is during our infancy, below the age of one (Erikson, 1950). Erikson argues that by feeding, the infant learns to trust, and by abandonment the infant learns to mistrust his/her mother as the primary attachment figure during the early years of life. While growing up and with an increasing action radius in our environment, we have repeated social encounters where we experience trust, betrayal of trust and mistrust. The positive and negative experiences shape a personal concept of how we understand trustworthiness and how we value trust for our relationships and engagement with others. Repeated positive trust experiences make it easier for us to trust others, whereas repeated experiences of mistrust and betrayal make us suspicious towards others. For the latter it will be more difficult to engage in new trust relationships. David Pilgrim and colleagues described the devastating effects of failure of trust in childhood. Abuse, overcritical parents, poor socio-economic family status or feeling the need to take care of parents all can lead to prolonged negative physical and mental health effects. Such negative experiences during early childhood and adolescence influence how those affected present themselves as patients, engage with medical professionals and build trust in medical professionals (Pilgrim, Tomasini and Vassilev, 2010).

Patient trust in doctors and, in some cases, individual trust in the wider health system develop during our personal encounters with health system professionals, and with the knowledge of existing health system guarantees such as regulations, accountability mechanisms or professional codes (Meyer et al, 2008). Often, health system professionals are seen as system representatives in the eyes of individuals, and when we trust our general practitioner, we are also more persuaded to trust the subsequent health system. The importance of health professionals for trust and public trust building must not be underestimated. Health professionals are the face of the health system and critical to trust building in general. In the American Midwest, a cross-sectional survey study with 142 participants evidently showed that patient trust in electronic health records is associated with 'patient trust in their primary care physician, patient recognition of the characteristics of EHRs, and patient perception of how the physician uses EHRs' (Qiao, Asan and Montague, 2015, p 360). The findings place the patient-doctor relationship in the spotlight for trust building.

While discussing personal experiences of trust and the experiences of others, public trust develops in the public sphere

(Gille, Smith and Mays, 2017). Public trust is a discourse-based construct shaped by a multitude of different actors. In the physical environment, trust-building discussions can take place when groups of people come together at work, in social and sport clubs and in the public space. We find such discourses in the online environment on social media platforms, online fora, and as part of the wider news media discourse as well. Examples of social media debates on different platforms such as Twitter, Facebook or Weibo about issues of trust include debates in the context of the COVID-19 pandemic in the Netherlands and Spain (Pérez-Escoda et al, 2020; van Dijck and Alinejad, 2020), maternal vaccination discourse and vaccine hesitancy during COVID-19 (Martin et al, 2020; Puri et al, 2020), organ donation consent legislation in Nova Scotia, Canada, or public opinion about organ donation in China (Xiong et al, 2021; Marcon et al, 2022). The present way in which we interact on social media platforms appears to form and dissolve communication strands around topical issues at a relatively fast pace. Using the example of Twitter, discussion emerges from general communication noise around hashtags, and once the issues are not of interest anymore to a wider audience, such discussion either morphs into evolving debates or disappears in Twitter archives. A Belgian study examining hashtags in the word cloud around #Coronavirus shows how numbers of tweets and retweets over time spike right after mass communications of COVID-19 related events of broad interest, such as jumps in infection or decisions to close schools (Kurten and Beullens, 2021). Such spikes are somewhat typical for the Twitter discourse and can be an indication of discourse spontaneously forming around hashtags. Unfortunately, the COVID-19 pandemic once again showcased that often social media debates and the discussion around certain topic areas are far from ideal, as the information discussed can be false and the social media platforms are viral spreaders of misinformation (Guntuku et al, 2021; Muric, Wu and Ferrara, 2021; Shahi, Dirkson and Majchrzak, 2021). Therefore, actors on the social media networks are responsible for acting upon the spread of misinformation (Limaye et al, 2020; Schillinger, Chittamuru and Ramírez, 2020). Corrections are a double-edged intervention against misinformation, as they can work but also can have counter-effects. Prior warnings on media platforms, reminders to check for accuracy and increased media literacy of the public can help to counteract misinformation (Borah, Irom and Hsu, 2021). Acknowledging the difficulty in assigning responsibilities to social media actors, as misinformation is not commonly defined and what some consider as misinformation others might understand as truthful information, several toolkits emerged to provide practical guidance on how to fight misinformation. Examples are the 2022 World Health Organization toolkit, *Toolkit for tackling misinformation on noncommunicable disease* (World Health Organization, 2022a), or the 2021 Office of the US Surgeon General, *Community Toolkit for Addressing Health Misinformation* (Office of the U.S. Surgeon General, 2021). At European Union level, major tech companies such as Google and Twitter signed the Code of Practice on Disinformation in 2018 (European Observatory on Health Systems and Policies, Fahy and Williams, 2021). In 2022, 37 international tech companies signed the self-regulatory 2022 Strengthened Code of Practice on Disinformation (European Commission, 2022b). The code covers several areas such as scrutiny of advertisement placements, political advertisement, platform integrity, empowerment of users, researchers and the fact checking community (European Commission, 2022a). How far such self-regulatory codes will be impactful in fighting misinformation will be seen in the future. Nevertheless, the emergence of different ways, such as toolkits as well as codes, to fight misinformation on different levels is a promising way forward. As truthful information is critical for trust building, the constant competition in social networks and media of misinformation and false information against true information is a persistent challenge for the trust-building discourse, which demands special attention if we want to build public trust (see Chapter Nine).

How misinformation and conspiracy threaten public trust building in the public sphere

Public trust develops in the public sphere where a wide range of actors communicate and discuss health system related information. Unfortunately, this discourse is often far from ideal and threatened by untruth and intentional spread of misinformation. There exists no common definition to describe misinformation (Krause et al, 2020). Broadly, misinformation can be understood in different ways, ranging from holding inaccurate beliefs with confidence to people's factual opinions that are unsupported by evidence and expert opinions (Vraga and Bode, 2020). As truthful information is desirable for the public trust-building discourse, conspiracy theories pose a particular problem as they not only influence conspiracy believers' trust in health care (Šuriņa et al, 2021), but also negatively influence levels of public trust with their false information (Goodnight and Poulakos, 1981; Papakostas, 2012; Oliver and T. J. Wood, 2014; Muirhead and Rosenblum, 2016).

In relation to the COVID-19 pandemic, in the German speaking part of Switzerland 10 per cent of the population strongly endorse conspiracy theories, and an additional 20 per cent of the population endorse conspiracy theories to some degree (Kuhn et al, 2021). Similar pictures appear in the United Kingdom, where 15 per cent of the population consistently and 10 per cent of the population strongly endorse conspiracy theories (Freeman et al, 2020), and in Croatia, where 23 per cent of the population strongly agree or agree with conspiracy theories (Tonković et al, 2021). Examples of such conspiracy theories are 'Bill Gates has created the virus in order to reduce the world population; Jews have created the virus to collapse the economy for financial gain; Lockdown is a way to terrify, isolate, and demoralize a society as a whole in order to reshape society to fit specific interests' (Kuhn et al, 2021, pp 7–8). Similarly to COVID-19 conspiracy theories, an array of medical conspiracy theories have developed over recent decades in relation to HIV/AIDS, MMR-vaccination, cholera, Ebola virus, polio virus, water fluoridation or phone use (Briggs, 2004; Oliver and T. Wood, 2014; Andrade, 2020; Bellatin et al, 2021). Despite the definition of conspiracy theory being contested, common features of such conspiracy theories are that 'the world or an event is held to be not as it seems; there is believed to be a cover-up by powerful others; the theory is accepted only by a minority; and the theory is unsupported by evidence' (Freeman et al, 2020, p 1). A wide range of psychological, epistemic, existential and social motives, as well as demographic and political factors, can influence people to believe in conspiracy theories (Douglas et al, 2019). What is particularly concerning is that conspiracy theories negatively influence conspiracy believers' engagement with health system activities, which translates to lower health and is linked to low levels of trust or mistrust in health system actors or the government being in charge of the health system (Brotherton, French and Pickering, 2013; Douglas et al, 2019; Jovančević and Milićević, 2020). Researchers agree that there is no doubt that levels of trust in health care and conspiracy theories in medicine influence each other. Different researchers describe the relationship of both concepts in different ways, but always with a negative outcome towards engagement with health care:

- trust as a mediator of conspiracy theories on behaviour (Bruder and Kunert, 2021);
- believing conspiracy theories lowers levels of trust (Krouwel et al, 2017; Mari et al, 2021);
- low levels of trust increases the likelihood of believing in conspiracy theories (Baier and Manzoni, 2020; Jovančević and Milićević, 2020); and

- strong distrust in official narratives can lead to believing contradicting conspiracy theories (Wood, Douglas and Sutton, 2012).

In addition to this close entanglement of trust and conspiracy theory, for both concepts, history and experience play an important role. Conspiracy theories often follow overarching (monological) belief systems that have strong historical roots (Goertzel, 1994; Swami et al, 2011; Mattocks et al, 2017; Douglas et al, 2019), and collective as well as personal experience influences levels of trust (Giddens, 1990; Luhmann, 2017). One example are the HIV/AIDS conspiracy beliefs and their influence on condom use and attitudes among the African American population. In 2005, both present conspiracy beliefs and mistrust leading to low rates of condom use were influenced by historic influences dating back to the Tuskegee syphilis study (conducted 1932–72) (Thomas and Quinn, 1991; Bogart and Thorburn, 2005; Bogart et al, 2010). While acknowledging that conspiracy theories or at least written evidence of conspiracy theories dates back to the 1320s and medieval history (McKenzie-McHarg, 2020), it appears that today's conspiracy theories often relate to a time frame somewhere between today and the 1930s/1940s. History is of particular importance as it has an impact on today's formation both of trust and conspiracy. Moreover, when reviewing conceptual research on conspiracy theory and comparing the work with conceptual work on trust, it is evident that both concepts share similarities when it comes to causes and effects. For example, fear, uncertainty, negative experience, discrimination, strong political ideology of the far left and right, all seem to lower levels of trust in the health system as well as increase the likelihood of believing in conspiracy theories. Equally, low trust and conspiracy theories share the same effect, that is, low or no participation with health system activities (Jolley and Douglas, 2014; Pummerer et al, 2021). From a conceptual viewpoint, despite research agreeing that trust and conspiracy theories are intertwined, little clarity exists that precisely conceptualises this relationship. This conceptual muddle undermines any meaningful attempt to increase conspiracy believers' trust, or to protect public trust from the influence of conspiracy theories. I argue that this knowledge gap not only threatens the health of the conspiracy believers' community (Oliver and T. Wood, 2014), but, considering their considerable size in some populations, might also negatively influence levels of public trust in health systems as conspiracy theorists diffuse conspiracy theories and false information into the public realm (Halpern et al, 2019). The need for conceptual clarification and research persists.

Public trust develops in the public sphere

While acknowledging the existence of conspiracy theories and misinformation, in an ideal scenario we can envision a public trust-building discourse that is open to all people. In this discourse, people can share their experiences with and thoughts about the health system. One suggestion of how such discourse can unfold is Jürgen Habermas' work on ideal speech situations and the public discourse in the public sphere. The ideal scenario of public trust-forming discourse is that all members of the public find themselves in a situation where:

1. 'Each subject who is capable of speech and action is allowed to participate in discourse.
2.
   (a) Each is allowed to call into question any proposal.
   (b) Each is allowed to introduce any proposal into the discourse.
   (c) Each is allowed to express his attitudes, wishes, and needs.
3. No speaker ought to be hindered by compulsion – whether arising inside the discourse or outside it – from making use of the rights secured under 1 and 2.' (White, 1990, p 56)

The arguments carried forward during debates in the ideal speech situation need to fulfil four validity criteria. They need to be comprehensible, true, authentic and morally right, and appropriate (Habermas, 1995; Gille, Smith and Mays, 2017). To build a consensus among the participants of such discourse all criteria of validity and ideal speech need to be met. This consensus–building process can lead to a common understanding of public trust.

Those situations of ideal speech are rare. There is no single public sphere where we all come together to discuss issues of trust, but a range of spheres form to discuss topics of public interest. Illustrated by the public debate about a wide range of COVID-19 issues, we can observe that issues of trust are discussed in a wide range of spheres with overlapping but also segregated population subgroups. This segregation is caused in part by our different preferences towards ways of communication, by cultural influences on how we communicate, by different personal views leading to the tendency that we might choose to engage with likeminded others, and accessibility hurdles that make it practically impossible to have an open access to all fora. Examples of such hurdles are mandatory subscription and registration requirements to be able to access certain fora, lack of digital skills and the digitalisation gaps in society more broadly, or social isolation. Nonetheless, what we read and with whom we discuss issues of trust on different platforms and within different spheres can shape public trust and our individual trust in a range of health system activities.

Building on earlier work of Evelien van der Schee (2016) and many examples of trust-building discourses in the public sphere, I propose a model that aims to describe how public trust develops (Schee, 2016; Gille, Smith and Mays, 2017, fig 2). Simplified, the model describes that public trust is a concept that develops from open public discourse in the public sphere as drawn in Figure 4.1. In the public sphere, private individuals and different actors from, within, and outside of the health system come together to discuss their own and

Figure 4.1: Simplified model to describe how public trust develops in the public sphere

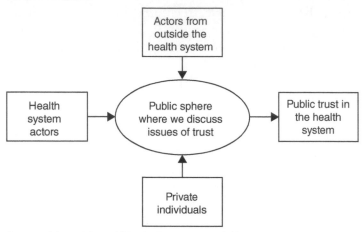

Source: Adapted from Gille, Smith and Mays 2017

others' experiences with health system activities. Examples of such discourse are discussions about COVID-19 contact tracing apps, vaccination or organ donation. During this discourse, we form a common understanding of what and whom we trust or do not trust. It is important to understand that the discourse is usually open to a wide range of actors and people with diverse interests and backgrounds. In my studies, analysing trust-building discourse in the NHS England context of data sharing for research and health system improvement, I found that members of the public make references to an astonishing range of actors from the local to the international level (Gille, 2017, chap 6). For example, for trust in the care. data program, members of the public understood that a very diverse group of actors influence trust, such as friends and family, journalists, campaigners, patient organisations, strangers, health care professionals, lawyers, researchers, advocates, private companies, the Department of Health, international technology companies, the European Union, and so on. This diversity of actors shows also that public trust grows within a discourse among a complex actors' network. The description of trust growing within a complex web of interactions is equally found in general trust-building models (Meyer et al, 2008). In a similar vein, several trust researchers constructed trust as a communication-based social phenomenon and public good. To this understanding, public trust hinges on active citizenship, democratic order, and its importance for social life in the public sphere (Fukuyama, 1995; Misztal, 1996; Seligman, 1997; Sztompka, 1999; O'Neill, 2002; Papakostas, 2012). What is particularly interesting is the view that public trust not only contributes to solidarity, toleration of others, and social cohesion by public discourse, but also builds the fundaments of democratic legitimacy similar to the concept of trust in politics (Misztal, 1996; Turper and Aarts, 2017). Legitimacy can be described as 'the capacity of a political system to engender and maintain the belief that existing political institutions are the most appropriate or proper ones for the society' (Lipset, 1959, p 86; Moodley, 2017). The concepts of public trust and legitimacy are often discussed in the context of legitimate data use for biobank research (O'Neill, 2002; Petersen, 2005), in the context of legal authority (Jackson and Gau, 2016), or political legitimacy (O'Sullivan, Healy and Breen, 2014); see Chapter Six. The interplay between public trust and legitimacy is a crucial outcome of trust building, as we like to see the activities in the health system to enjoy public legitimacy.

Concluding remarks

Private individuals and actors from within and outside the health system come together in the public sphere to discuss issues of trust. This public discourse forms public trust. Since there is no single public sphere, we see these discussions emerging simultaneously in different fora and on different platforms. Public trust building depends on truthful information and therefore intentional misinformation and conspiracy theories threaten the public trust–building process. To contribute to public trust building, credible health care professionals and health policy makers need to engage in the public sphere to convey truthful information and to engage in public dialogue. If health care professionals do not engage with and enter the public information space, it is upon others to fill this space, whether they are a reliable, credible and a knowledgeable information source or not.

FIVE

What builds public trust?

Health system actors can build and destroy public trust with their words and actions. Trust research focuses on dynamics of trust and suggests what actions can build trust in a specific context. When comparing studies investigating public trust, it becomes obvious that there exists no universally applicable blueprint for public trust building. This is not surprising as trust is context specific. In the context of public trust in data use in the health system, 13 themes describe what the public understands to be important for public trust building (Gille, Smith and Mays, 2020). These themes form an important part of the public trust concept discussed in this book and provide the basis for the subsequent chapters. The themes in Table 5.1 are at a level of abstraction where they do not overlap in content and are detailed enough to provide a meaningful representation of the data they emerged from. They are presented in alphabetical order, as there is no ranking of importance for the trust-building process associated with the themes. The themes are grouped according to their main time reference: past, present, and future. The threefold categorisation reflects on the one hand the basic principles of trust building based on past experiences, present perceptions, and future anticipations; on the other hand, it provides some preliminary guidance for

Table 5.1: Themes building public trust in the health system

Time reference	Themes	Explanations in terms of 'if, then' statements
Past	Familiarity	If people have positive experiences with the actor, then people trust more.
Present	Active regulatory systems	If regulatory systems are in place, then people trust more.
	Anonymity	If private data is anonymised before sharing, then people trust more.
	Autonomy	If health system actors enable people to maintain autonomy, then people trust more.
	Gut feeling	If people's gut feeling 'tells' them to trust, then people trust more.
	Information quality	If truthful and honest information is provided, then people trust more.
	Privacy	If people's privacy is maintained, then people trust more.
	Potential	If a potential to fulfil the purpose for why trust is established is recognised, then people trust more.
	Respect	If the public and actors respect each other, then people trust more.
	Security	If action is perceived to be secure, then people trust more.
Future	Certainty about the future	If researchers and officials do the best they can do to foresee risk in the future, then people trust more.
	Net benefit	If a net benefit (benefit to others, health system benefit, personal benefit, public financial benefit) occurs, then people trust more.
	Time	If action is not rushed, then people trust more.

Source: Adapted from Gille, Smith and Mays 2020

trust-building activities as discussed in Part III of this book. Namely that public trust not only comprises a range of themes, but also sits within a time continuum between the past and the future. Niklas Luhmann wrote that a theory of time is imperative for a theory of trust, as trust is a future-oriented construct which allows us to act as if we are somewhat certain about the future (Luhmann, 2017). Further, we can identify the themes that are a) distinctive for public trust, and b) distinctive for the context of data use in health care. The anticipation of a net benefit is somewhat specific for health system activities that particularly depend on public trust, as the trusted health system action has altruistic components leading to the benefit for others. We consent to the research use of our electronic health record with the motivation that the findings of this research might help others and future society. Themes that are typical to describe trust in health data use are anonymity, privacy and security. All three contribute to data confidentiality and privacy protection. When reading the list of themes and the following explanations, you will notice that most themes are intuitive to understand and reflect our personal trust experiences as private individuals. This is not unexpected as individual trust is the underlying construct of public trust. Individuals form the public and we all have a personal understanding of what trust means to us.

Theme relating to the past

One theme, familiarity, relates to past personal experiences that influence public trust building in the present. Other research suggests that the theme familiarity can be expanded beyond personal experiences to include experiences of others and collective memory (Ferrera et al, 2016). Studies on trust in insurance companies show that a loyal family history with an insurance company can influence children's trust in the same insurance company of their parents (Natalier and Willis, 2008). Similarly, we place initial trust in a new general practitioner because s/he was recommended by friends and family based on their positive experiences. In a bigger historical context, over 30 years after the German reunification, we can observe an East-West rift wherein East Germans have less trust in regulatory and representative institutions as compared to West Germans. The reasons may be found somewhere between the autocratic past of former East Germany and the unification process itself (Braun and Trüdinger, 2022). Recent anecdotal evidence from my ongoing research shows how strong historical impacts on society inform present trust building in digital health activities: in the summer of 2022, in Hall in Tirol, Austria, a local citizen described to me that the city psychiatric hospital and nursing home was part of Adolf Hitler's Euthanasia Program Aktion T-4. A commission from Berlin used patient records to select 360 patients to be deported and murdered in the Tötungsanstalten (Killing Facilities) Hartheim and Niedernhart in Austria (Deutscher Paritätischer Wohlfahrtsverband, Landesverband Berlin e.V., 2022). Therefore, s/he was suspicious towards the present electronic health record program in Austria. Such suspicion can influence how we interact with health care providers (Mechanic, 1998). This example raises an important issue, namely that negative experiences, even those of our ancestors, have a strong influence on parts of the public and are particularly difficult to overcome. I argue it would be foolish to ignore such fears merely because from the present expert viewpoint, current electronic health data collection activities are based on fundamentally different motivations, laws and understanding of ethics. On the contrary, it is important to address such beliefs to overcome history-motivated suspicion and mistrust.

Familiarity

Previous positive experiences with the health system are a fundament for trust. This fact is not specific to health system settings and is very intuitive for trust building (Sztompka,

1998). Shared positive experiences are an especially strong basis for mutual trust. The importance of positive experiences explains why for some actors a long-term reputation is so valuable, and why a reputation loss and negative experiences with the health system can drastically lower levels of trust. Because previous experiences are unchangeable, present actions contributing to trust building are important, as today's actions will be the past experiences of tomorrow.

Themes relating to the present

Nine trust-building themes largely relate to the present. These themes are active adherence to regulation, anonymisation of personal data, offering autonomous choices to the public, a gut feeling that motivates to place trust, truthful and honest information about a health system activity, protecting privacy, showing a potential to be able to fulfil the trusted action, respectful interaction with health data and the public, and keeping data secure. In comparison with familiarity and themes relating to the future, this set of themes might feel more implementable and easier to approach as they relate to our present actions. But this does not suggest that these themes are more important.

Active regulatory systems

When health system actors adhere to law and regulation, the public is more likely to trust such actors. Adherence to law and regulation is a commonly identified trust-building theme. Law and regulatory systems can be understood as system guarantees for trustworthy behaviour (Meyer et al, 2008). Complying with law is critical for data sharing activities in health systems (National Data Guardian, 2020). When we know that a health data activity in the health system context is bound to health data regulation and law, we are more inclined to trust this activity (Milne et al, 2019). Having said that, for those being critical towards the content and intention of some health data legislation, adherence to legislation can be less important for trust building.

Trust in the existence of regulatory systems is framed by the bigger context of trust in the legislative power itself and trust in the appropriate use and application of the respective legislation. Laws and regulations are fundamental for trustworthy data use in health systems, but equally important is the appropriate adherence to and implementation of legislation by health system actors.

Anonymity

In the context of data sharing, as for example making electronic health records available for research in precision medicine or health system improvement, the public likes to see that their data is anonymised to be able to trust the data–sharing process. The usual logic behind the wish for anonymity is that parts of the public understand anonymity to protect their privacy. Unfortunately, there exists a knowledge gap among some members of the public about the capacity of anonymity to protect privacy, as well as what degrees of anonymity are used in research. In the context of the care.data initiative in England, some members of the public demanded complete anonymity, as in 100 per cent, to trust the use of health data for health system management and research (Gille and Brall, 2021b). Such a rigorous expectation towards anonymity is neither realistic nor feasible in practice. Some in the research community have highlighted for years that anonymity, for example in the context of genetic research, is increasingly difficult to maintain and donors are potentially identifiable (Lunshof et al, 2008). The reason is that with the advancement of big data analytics it will become impossible to guarantee full anonymity. Therefore, anonymity is not the ideal solution to privacy (Savage, 2016). The crux for public trust building is that if parts of the public place trust in data sharing based on a mistaken understanding of the capabilities of anonymity to protect their privacy, such trust is inherently flawed and at risk of being damaged. It is necessary to equip the public with a sufficient understanding of the relationship between anonymity and privacy, as well as what privacy-maintaining mechanisms exist in practice aside from anonymity. An informed understanding of anonymity and realistic expectations towards anonymity are important for the public to discuss in an informed way issues of trustworthy data-sharing activities in health systems. Considering the impact of digitalisation on society, such knowledge will also become useful outside of health system activities.

Autonomy

Being able to make one's own choices in the health system builds trust in the health system. To exercise this autonomy, such choices need to be offered to the public by the health system. Anchored in deeper theoretical descriptions of trust, the possibility to choose between alternatives is a cornerstone of trust building. Following Luhmann, in situations of choice we place trust as we choose one alternative over the other (Luhmann, 2017). Where there is no choice, we hope for a better outcome or have confidence in the wider system; see Chapter Two. One example of such exercised autonomy is the data control which can support trust building in mobile health applications (Butt et al, 2022).

An important debate evolved in recent years about different consent models for electronic health records and organ donations (Shepherd, O'Carroll and Ferguson, 2014; Chan et al, 2016). Should members of the public take part in these activities by default, and if they revoke consent opt-out, or should members of the public voluntarily opt-in? From a trust-building perspective, some favour asking the public to consent (opt-in) to electronic health records, others advocate for an opt-out model. We see that both models are used. Arguments for opt-out are early benefit for patients, reduced workload and less bureaucracy. Arguments for opt-in are acknowledgement of patient control, ownership and autonomy (Watson and Halamka, 2006). Real-world examples show that opt-out models for the introduction of nationwide electronic health record systems are successful in some countries and fail in others. It is important to engage the public and health system actors with public consultations in the planning process of such activities, and communicate to the public in an appropriate way about the health system activity; see Chapter Nine (Meszaros, Ho and Corrales Compagnucci, 2020).

Gut feeling

Gut feeling is the only retrospectively added theme to this concept, as gut feeling was not represented in the qualitative data from the three case studies of my research. Instead, this theme represents a body of literature that describes how trust building is motivated by emotions (Engdahl and Lidskog, 2014). Michael Calnan and Rosemary Rowe, in their seminal work on trust in health care, describe that trust comprises of cognitive elements and affective dimension (Calnan and Rowe, 2008). For some it might be difficult to describe why we trust, it just feels right. All other themes in this concept might feel to them synthetic. In fact, when combing the present trust research landscape, including the many guidelines that explain how one can be trustworthy and eventually build trust, as for example seen among the ethics and trust guidelines of artificial intelligence (Jobin, Ienca and Vayena, 2019), we can easily come to the conclusion that trust building is a calculated process following an analytical paradigm. As if we have a checklist in our head representing the themes discussed here, and when a certain number of boxes are ticked, we trust. This calculated approach to trust building certainly makes it easier for policy makers and other health system actors to tailor their trust-building actions, but this approach might be insufficient as it neglects emotions. Other researchers suggested the concept of intuitive trust to describe this form of trust building (Dane, Rockmann and Pratt, 2012).

Information quality

Communication of information about the to-be-trusted is significant to the trust-building process (Fukuyama, 1995; Larson, 2016). A five-year comparison on patient-centered communication in China shows the importance of high-quality information and reliable information sources for trust building (Liu and Jiang, 2021). Understandable information, from a reliable person, that we view as honest and truthful builds trust. The same is true for online health information (Wang, Shi and Kong, 2021). We tend to trust when several information sources agree and provide similar if not the same information. This vital need of information for trust building explains in part the rise in research examining the relationship of transparency with trust, as well as the general societal call for more political transparency within and outside of health system governance (Stafford, Cole and Heinz, 2022). For example, in biomedical research, transparent governance processes are anticipated to build public trust in data sharing (Gille, Axler and Blasimme, 2020). Similarly, researchers suggest that transparency of data governance and data use builds public trust in secondary use of health data and data science more broadly (Ford et al, 2019; Meszaros and Ho, 2019). Yet, transparency strategies need to be meaningful and purpose driven to have an effect on public trust (Banner, 2022).

Privacy

Together with security and anonymity, privacy is one of the key themes contributing to trust in health data use. Most of us value our privacy and would like to see that privacy protection mechanisms are in place when health data is used and shared (Damschroder et al, 2007; McGraw et al, 2009; Thapa and

Camtepe, 2021; Townsend, 2022; Degerli, 2023). Privacy can be understood as the appropriate use of user's information. Multiple factors contribute to privacy, ranging from policy aspects focusing on use and purpose, legislation, technological aspects and Privacy by Design, to human behaviour and social mechanisms (Schaar, 2010; Fang et al, 2017; Abouelmehdi, Beni-Hessane and Khaloufi, 2018). Privacy by Design follows the approach that privacy preserving mechanisms are built into the design of the technology and not added retrospectively (Duncan, 2007).

Potential

We need to see the potential of a health system activity or actor to achieve what we would like to trust it. We will not place trust in something or someone we consider as not being able to fulfil the to-be-trusted action. Such potential develops, among other sources, from the healthy self-confidence of an actor and reputation; by showing a track record of accomplishments; from skills and education which lead to conclusions about the actor's abilities to complete a task in a trusted way; the impression that a health system activity is well structured and planned; and, that the health system activity is designed based on the latest knowledge in the field.

Respect

We do not trust someone who we perceive as disrespectful. The same is true if we see that our data is not treated with respect. Respectful data interaction requires that actors working with data do not lose data or work inaccurately with data, leading to the introduction of false and incomplete data sets. Data must not be leaked or disclosed to others without consent. The notion of respect for trust building in health care is widely recognised in research and commonly accepted

(O'Neill, 2002; Gilson, 2003; Mohseni and Lindstrom, 2007; Østergaard, 2015).

Security

Security mechanisms to safeguard health data contribute to trust building (Ostherr et al, 2017; Muller et al, 2021; Kalkman et al, 2022). For example, trust linked to the degree of data security, next to privacy, quality, and processing of data, is important for the acceptance of mobile health diabetes self-management apps (Schretzlmaier, Hecker and Ammenwerth, 2022). Data security is an integral part of health data systems and digital health applications. Also, health data governance principles that guide data collection, storage, use and sharing cover data security aspects to assure a trustworthy data environment (Rosenbaum, 2010). In ethics review processes for big data research, considerations of data security are part of ethics proposal evaluations (Ienca et al, 2018). In the debate about cyber threats and hacking, data security is a frontrunner for trust building (Coventry and Branley, 2018). Despite the fact that many data security aspects are technology based, it is the responsibility of all health system actors to contribute to overall health system safety (Kohn, Corrigan and Donaldson, 2000).

Themes relating to the future

Three themes describe future aspects of public trust: certainty about the future, anticipation of a net benefit as an outcome of the trust relationship, and time given to those who work with the entrusted data. Linking the public trust concept to the future is important as the nature of trust is future facing. We build trust based on past experiences, present perceptions and future anticipations, but the outcome of a trust relationship will always come into effect in the future. We only get confirmation if our trust is justified after the previously expected outcome becomes reality.

Certainty about the future

The inability to foresee the future is one of the reasons why trust is required. If we could foresee the future and know the outcome of present actions, trust would be in most cases a useless construct. Trust being a future-oriented construct, it has the capacity to overcome the uncertainty of the future unknown, and allows us to act as if we have an understanding of the future (Luhmann, 2017). We usually trust when we have a perception of assurances of future beneficial outcomes (Simpson, 2007). When we place trust, we would like to know how the trusted action will unfold. Health system activities need to have inbuilt processes to keep the anticipated outcome of such activities in focus. Knowledge about the mechanisms and processes in place to meet targets helps to make judgements about the likelihood that anticipated outcomes become reality. Such processes are, for example, interim evaluations, accountability and oversight structures, transparency and communication strategies, quality control and audits (Deschênes and Sallée, 2005; Vollmer et al, 2018; Blasimme and Vayena, 2020; O'Neill, 2020).

Net benefit

We trust in anticipation of a beneficial outcome as a result of our trust relationship with the health system (Platt and Kardia, 2015; Platt, Raj and Kardia, 2019). We will not place trust when we anticipate a negative outcome. Betrayed trust can have negative consequences for us and others. The same is true for trust which was based on misinformation and false judgements of trustworthiness. We place trust in the first instance with the anticipation of a benefit, or at least no harm. Depending on the health system activity we trust in, we can identify a range of benefits as an outcome of a trust relationship. These benefits are, for example: a) benefit to others, b) personal benefit, c) health system benefit and

d) public financial benefit. We trust a vaccination to protect us and others from vaccine-preventable diseases. We weigh the potential privacy risks against anticipated benefits when we accept electronic health records systems (Li et al, 2014). We share our data for medical research trusting that the outcome of this research will not only lead to improved quality of care, but also financial gains that are beneficial to the overall health system. We trust a medical app to personally benefit our health and trust that the collected information might help other app users to optimise their health (Haasteren et al, 2019).

The anticipation of a net benefit requires health system actors to show to the public what these benefits are. If health communication cannot show the anticipated benefits of a specific health system action, it is unlikely that the public will place trust in the health system activity.

Time

Time has at least two implications for trust building. On the one hand, we need time to decide if we want to trust and therefore trust building should not be rushed; on the other hand, those who are trusted should take their time to complete what they are trusted for. Time is a reccurring theme in trust in health care research, especially during the decision making process within patient-doctor relationships and the wish of patients that doctors spend enough time with them (Keating et al, 2004; Levine, 2004; Schee et al, 2007; Shaya et al, 2019). The time-dependence of trust has implications for policy making and health system governance, in that it demands policy processes that are not hurried to allow the public to build trust. However, there appears to be a fine balance between providing enough time to grow public trust and designing health policy with a reasonable implementation time frame. In my present research on public trust in national electronic health records, preliminary unpublished evidence from small group discussions with German citizens suggests that an implementation strategy of a national electronic health record system which is perceived by the public as too slow undermines trust. The argument is that excessively slow health policy implementation can appear as unprofessional and ill-managed.

Concluding remarks

This chapter presented 13 public trust-building themes. The themes were grouped along a time continuum from past and present to the future. Twelve themes were developed from qualitative data and one theme, gut feeling, originated from theory to represent the body of literature that shows how trust develops from motivations and feelings as opposed to calculated decisions. Distinctive themes of public trust in data use are themes relating to privacy, security and anonymity. The anticipation of a net benefit is a considerably more distinctive theme of public trust as compared to individual trust.

SIX

What are the effects of public trust?

Health system legitimisation and public acceptance are the results of a strong public-system trust relationship. Participation and legitimisation are fundamental to the success of health system activities and explain why we care about high levels of public trust (Misztal, 1996). In the wide breadth of health system activities, we anticipate that participation translates into improved levels of population health. When considering a democratic understanding of the public-state relationship, we like to see that health system activities enjoy public legitimisation. Public trust is by no means the only reason why we participate in health system activities, and health system legitimisation does not exclusively develop from public trust. However, both effects are crucial to the public trust concept and explain why public trust in health systems is essential for population health.

Participation

When we trust, we engage in, participate in or accept a trusted action. Alternative terms to participation are buy-in, acceptance, adoption, engagement, co-production or consent. Positive experiences within the health system usually build trust in the health system. This is a very intuitive and commonly known effect of trust experienced outside of health systems, which we also experience in our private life, in relationships with friends, among colleagues and business partners. In the context of health systems, a survey study conducted in 2021 in South Dakota showed positive and statistically significant effects of trust in government and trust in physicians on the probability of COVID-19 vaccine uptake (Viskupič, Wiltse and Meyer, 2022). A 2021 survey study in Iran presented similar results showing that generalised trust and trust in the health system are positively associated with the willingness to get vaccinated against COVID-19 (Ahorsu et al, 2022). A 2021 multi-country survey study from Asia also found that high levels of public trust in the government are associated with the adoption of COVID-19 vaccination certificates. Interestingly, the authors suggest that low levels of trust in COVID-19 vaccination might have a negative effect on trust in COVID-19 vaccination certificates (Kc et al, 2022). Such spill effects can occur in two ways. First, when trust spills over from trust in individuals to trust in institutions. Second, when trust spills over from one institution to another institution or activity, which usually happens when different health system activities are associated with the same actor, for example government (Suh, Chang and Lim, 2012; Høyer and Mønness, 2016). Accordingly, low levels of trust in the political system can spill over to low levels of trust in the health system, as witnessed in the context of the Ebola crisis in Sierra Leone (Ozawa, Paina and Qiu, 2016). Spill-over effects should remind us to look beyond a specific context and to consider the broader societal as well as system context when examining public trust.

Trust is also critical for the adoption of new technologies in health care and society in general. Luhmann argued that, with the technological development of societies, trust will become increasingly important (Luhmann, 2017). Examples of new technologies in health systems that are dependent on sufficient levels of public trust to succeed include the acceptance of e-government applications; the use of artificial intelligence applications in health care; the use of mobile health devices such as fitness tracker wearables; the adoption of electronic health records or electronic vaccination certificates; the introduction of health data cooperatives; the involvement in decision making on health data use, reuse, access and sharing; or the public acceptance of larger health data spaces open for public and private research activities (Warkentin et al, 2002; Hafen, Kossmann and Brand, 2014; Hays and Daker-White, 2015; Haasteren et al, 2019; Nundy, Montgomery and Wachter, 2019; Ienca and Vayena, 2020; Gille and Vayena, 2021; Nwebonyi, Silva and de Freitas, 2022; Samuel et al, 2022).

Closely linked to engagement with the health system by members of the public is the growth of social capital and cohesion within societies. Social capital grows by means of collaborative action to achieve common goals (Gilson, 2003). Social capital itself is not commonly defined, but in the context of public trust in the health system, social capital can be understood as 'a person's or group's sympathy toward another person or group that may produce a potential benefit, advantage, and preferential treatment for another person or group of persons beyond that expected in an exchange relationship' (Robison, Schmid and Siles, 2002, p 19). Increased levels of social capital lead to social stability, prosperity, happiness and health (Fukuyama, 1995; Nieminen et al, 2013).

Public trust leads to participation in health system activities. By engaging with others, public trust builds social capital. Both effects are important for the health system and society as they lead to improved levels of health.

Legitimisation

Next to the effect of public trust on participation, public trust also legitimises health system activities. Legitimacy is often associated with trust in politics or institutions (Weatherford, 1992). Legitimacy can be understood as 'a belief that a governing institution has the right to rule and exercises this

right appropriately' (Dellmuth et al, 2022, p 11). In the context
of health system activities, such as the introduction of national
electronic health record systems, this means that when the
public trusts the health system to use electronic health records,
the health system has the legitimacy to do so. Furthermore,
public trust is critical to maintain the health system and protect
it from disintegration (Noyon, de Keijser and Crijns, 2020).
In democratic societies, government legitimacy develops from
public trust translated into votes during election processes
and the rotation of parties in government (Misztal, 1996).
Alternatively, legitimacy can develop from a public trust-based
social contract/licence between the public and the government
(Hardin, 2009; Levine, 2019). A social license can be described
as an agreement between the public and the government or
health system actor, such as a biobank, to operate in accordance
with societal normative expectations (Parsons and Moffat, 2014;
Gehman, Lefsrud and Fast, 2017; Gille, Vayena and Blasimme,
2020). A 2021 study in the Portuguese context supports that
trust in political institutions reinforces health policy legitimacy
(Asensio, 2021). During the COVID-19 pandemic, several studies
researched trust and legitimacy of COVID-19 health policies and
interventions (Bekker, Ivankovic and Biermann, 2020; Giritli
Nygren and Olofsson, 2021; Hanson et al, 2021). Aside from the
COVID-19 context, studies in the context of data use in health
systems and governments broadly support the important link of
trust and legitimacy (Moodley, 2017; Mensah and Adams, 2020).
Similarly, it is important that health system activities enjoy public
legitimacy to ensure that the public takes part in health system
activities. If the public loses trust, the public also withdraws
public legitimacy, which can lead to a stagnation of health system
activities or insufficient use of resources (Misztal, 1996).

Concluding remarks

Participation and legitimacy are the main effects of public trust.
Both are important for the health system to work successfully.

SEVEN

What frames public trust?

Knowledge about the context is key to successful public trust building. An accurate understanding of the context of public trust is the first important step towards a meaningful development of a conceptual framework (Schee et al, 2007; Kaasa and Andriani, 2022). This chapter provides an overview of context-related themes framing public trust. The previous two chapters described what builds public trust and what the effect of public trust is. Both sets of themes are important to describe what public trust is as they describe the cause and effect of public trust. However, we need additional information about what frames the concept. The themes discussed in this chapter provide richer information about the context the public trust concept works in. The nine themes in Table 7.1 provide insights into issues that can heavily influence the concept or are a prerequisite for public trust growth. We see that often such framing themes are neglected in debates about public trust or considered as marginally important for the development of public trust. However, these themes are critical for the successful build-up of public trust, or when the public trust-building themes fail, we might find the reason among the framing themes.

Table 7.1: Framing themes of public trust in the health system

Level of application	*Framing themes*	Explanation
Generic	*Communication*	We need to communicate to build trust.
	Reason for the need of public trust	We need a reason to trust.
	Risk	We cannot get around risks in trust relationships.
Individual	*Fear*	To fear is a human characteristic.
	Human error	Humans make errors and a trust relationship should endure human error.
	World-view	Our world-view shapes the wider understanding of trust.
	Religion and afterlife	Our religious beliefs can influence the decision to trust.
Public	*Public mood*	The public mood can influence our perception of trustworthiness.
Government	*Trust cannot be expected*	Expectation on the part of those with political power to enjoy public trust by default is noxious.

Source: Adapted from Gille, Smith and Mays 2020

The themes are sorted in four levels mirroring the model of how public trust develops in the public sphere; see Chapter Four (Gille, Smith and Mays, 2017). Generic themes are fundamental for public trust to work. Themes at the individual, public and government level are foremost associated with the respective actor level. This helps to locate the framing themes among the actors involved in the public trust–building process and guides appropriate action to deal with the framing themes, if needed.

Communication

Communication is the bedrock of public trust. We will only build public trust when we communicate with each other and thereby exchange information about each other. If we have no information about the to-be-trusted other, we will not be able to place trust. As described in Chapter Two, communication needs to be understood in three different ways: a) exchanging words, b) recognising signals and signs, and c) processing personal and collective experiences in our memories during the trust-building process. The information needs to be truthful to build public trust. Chapter Nine describes in greater detail how communication can foster public trust.

Reason for the need of public trust

We need a reason to trust. In the health system context, we place trust because we anticipate a benefit as the result of the trusted action. If we do not need such a benefit or do not want to take part in a health system activity, public trust will not emerge. Even generalised trust, a somewhat diffuse form of trust in society, might appear initially to not be focused on a specific reason, nevertheless it has a purpose as it helps to deal with the overall uncertainty of life. Generalised trust makes it easier to engage with strangers and is a considerable variable for social capital (Bjørnskov, 2007; Stolle, 2015). Probably every form of trust is established for a reason that can be specified to a varying degree.

Risk

Trusting is an inherently risky activity as trust can be betrayed and misused (Bohnet and Zeckhauser, 2004; Smith, 2017). For many, trust is a bet 'about the future uncertain and uncontrollable actions of others' (Sztompka, 1999, p 31). Health system activities themselves carry risks, for example financial risks as well as risks of technical or information system failure (Murray and Frenk, 2000; Narayana Samy, Ahmad and Ismail, 2010). Both sources of risk, on the one hand the risk of betrayal and on the other hand health system risks, make the trusting party vulnerable towards negative outcomes of the trust relationship. Patients and the public have an expectation towards the health system to not be betrayed, and the health system tries to mitigate risks where possible, but there is no guarantee of a risk-free health system.

Fear

To fear is human. Patient fears and anxieties are well known to health professionals. During the 2014–15 Ebola outbreak in Sierra Leone, fears relating to a lack of trust in the Ebola response system delayed care seeking (Yamanis, Nolan and Shepler, 2016). Public fears that lead to counterproductive behaviour need to be addressed (May, 2005). A qualitative study in England identified five public fears about data sharing, which are: '(1) inadequate security and exploitation, (2) data inaccuracy, (3) distrust, (4) discrimination and inequality, and (5) less patient-centered care' (Lounsbury et al, 2021, p 9). As the examples show, fears can prolong treatment and inhibit engagement with health care. Trust theory describes fears as a serious hazard to trust building (O'Neill, 2003; Pilgrim, Tomasini and Vassilev, 2010). From a sequential trust-building viewpoint, fears usually sit at the very front and block the start of the trust-building process. Health system actors and health system communication strategies need to address such fears to create an environment where those who fear feel comfortable to interact with the health system.

Human error

To err is human and errors are costly for the health system as they burn trust (Kohn, Corrigan and Donaldson, 2000;

Jacobs, 2005). Despite the constant and of utmost importance drive to improve health systems and prevent errors, it is probably impossible to run a health system free from error (Bleetman et al, 2012). Measures to reduce errors are, for example, computerised medication order entry systems and the use of electronic health records (Bates et al, 1999; Middleton et al, 2013). To allow trust to build in such an environment, a realistic expectation of the public towards the health system is necessary, as an expectation of an error-free health system unfortunately cannot yet be fulfilled. At the same time, when patients maintain trust in health system processes that are error laden and have considerable safety problems, they make themselves highly vulnerable towards these errors (Entwistle and Quick, 2006). The complexity of the relationship between trust and human errors is difficult to solve. On the one hand, human errors harm trust. On the other hand, the expectation of an error-free health system to build trust is difficult to accomplish, and last, false trust in high-error health system processes exposes patients to high risks. Constant health system improvement, the awareness that human errors are unfortunately occurring and attention to such errors when building trust can be a way forward to build trust while acknowledging the possibility of human errors.

World-view

People's attitudes towards life and their world-view influence their trust-building behaviour. Based on their education, culture and experience, people build assumptions about the world (Koltko-Rivera, 2004). These assumptions determine people's behaviour. For example, axioms such 'what can be done, will be done' express a disillusioned attitude towards data use in the care.data context (Gille, Smith and Mays, 2020). In a recent interview study on trustworthy data use in health systems, a participant told me that adherence to legislation and regulation is less important for trust building, as many examples exist where health system actors breached the law and were still fully functioning. Such disappointment is a hurdle that needs to be overcome before trust can be built. In contrast, positive mindsets and attitudes can build resilience and contribute to community building and engagement in times of crisis (Van den Broucke, 2020).

Religion and afterlife

Religion can have a strong effect on public perceptions of health system activities and trust building. A 1998 study among 1,274 adults in the US showed that religiously active people have higher levels of trust in their physicians (Benjamins, 2006). In contrast, and with a different focus, a 2005 survey with 1,200 participants in the US found 'that religion still remains the most important factor in fostering public reservations about emerging technologies, particularly the stem cell controversy, after we control all other variables' (Liu and Priest, 2009, p 715). Religious leaders can also have a strong influence on health care engagement and acceptance of health system interventions among religious communities (Chu, Pink and Willer, 2021). Like fears, religious beliefs can influence upfront how parts of the public engage with health system activities. In a similar notion, spiritual beliefs and beliefs about what happens after someone's death can impact trust building in health system activities such as organ donation, or data use for research purposes (Cheung, Alden and Wheeler, 1998; Newton, 2011; Gille and Brall, 2021a). To build trust in settings where religious beliefs and beliefs about afterlife are hindering trust building, it is important to address such beliefs and to create space for religious beliefs in health system activities; see Chapter Nine.

Public mood

Many societies were shaken in recent years by a series of national and international events with a severe negative impact on public sentiment towards national and international governments. Such events included the 2008 global financial crisis; the 2015 Syrian refugee crisis; the 2019 COVID-19 pandemic; the withdrawal of the United Kingdom from the European Union (Brexit) in 2020; the global climate crisis; nationalist movements, political movements against the rule of law in some European countries, and questions about European identity (Jenkins, 2008; Altomonte, 2019; Alhaffar and Janos, 2021). Such a crises series introduces instability and uncertainty into societies, which might explain why trust evolved in recent years into a topic of broader interest. As trust has the capacity to mitigate uncertainty, the public feels the need to discuss and establish trust. However, trust is prone to spill over effects, and therefore low levels of trust in the government can spill from one crisis to the other (Montinola, 2004). A history of bad governmental crises management does not build public trust in new crises management capabilities. Such suspicion of the government threatens trust (O'Neill, 2003).

Trust cannot be expected

Trust grows freely and can neither be enforced nor expected (Misztal, 1996). If parts of the government expect to be trusted by the public, they undermine public trust and harm fundamental democratic principles (Gille, Smith and Mays, 2020). Health system actors and policy makers need to work towards earning public trust and do their best to contribute to trust building. There are no shortcuts, and bypassing trust-building activities with the motivation to save time will likely fail.

Concluding remarks

The set of nine framing themes discussed in this chapter shows the complex nature of contextual factors that can influence public trust building in a positive and/or negative way. The set of themes provides an overview of what health policy makers and health system professionals should consider when building public trust.

PART III

How can we foster public trust in the health system?

If we agree that public trust is important for well-functioning health systems, in its capacity to lead to public participation in health system activities as well as to legitimise health system activities, we need ways to maintain public trust or to build public trust where necessary. Summarised in the list presented later, I propose three areas as the keys to cultivating public trust: a) governance and policy actions that aim to build public trust, Chapter Eight; b) communication strategies that convey trustworthiness and repair trust if broken, Chapter Nine; and c), monitoring public trust, Chapter Ten. Informed by the conceptual work presented in Part II of this book, careful governance and health policy making with an eye on public trust are important, as they should lead to trustworthy health care activities and thereafter lead to the establishment of public trust. To build trust we need to convey truthful information about what makes someone or something trustworthy. Without communication we cannot establish public trust. Last, we want to evaluate if our trust-building governance and health policy making led to the anticipated effect of establishing public trust in health system activities. To evaluate our performance, we need to be able to collect reliable data about public trust. By collecting data about public trust, we can make conclusions about the effectiveness of a health policy and can inform health system improvement, policy making and health system reforms. The combination of the three public trust-building areas provides a wide spectrum of activities that are promising to build public trust. The following three points offer high-level guidance on how to build public trust, and the subsequent chapters substantiate these points with applied examples linked to the conceptual framework of this book.

Actions needed to build public trust in the health system are:

1. Develop a comprehensive understanding of public trust in the health system activity of focus.
2. Derive from point one:
    a. policy and governance actions that build public trust.
    b. communication strategies that build public trust.
    c. methods to collect reliable data about public trust.
3. Collect data about public trust and evaluate if the public trust-building actions meet their targets.

EIGHT

How can we build public trust by means of effective health policy and governance?

Around the globe, health systems are complex systems in which a variety of actors contribute to a wide range of health care activities and processes. From a citizen perspective, such health care processes can be exemplified in five consecutive steps, which are: a) keeping the public healthy with preventive mechanisms such as vaccination programmes; b) reaching out proactively to detect health problems; c) diagnosing diseases; d) treating diseases; and e) providing good end of life care (Bergman, Neuhauser and Provost, 2011). To operate a health system to the best of its abilities, as well as to provide high quality care to patients and the public, access, storage, and use of health data is fundamental. Health data is not only used for routine health care operations and health system management, but also for biomedical research, the development of new medical technologies and public health research more broadly (Weber, Mandl and Kohane, 2014; Milne et al, 2019; Gille, Vayena and Blasimme, 2020). The collection and use of health data in nationally and internationally coordinated ways hinges on a range of technical, legal, ethical and societal issues, among which public trust in health data use is considered by many as a corner-stone (Ostherr et al, 2017; Lawler et al, 2018; Vayena and Blasimme, 2018; Heijlen and Crompvoets, 2021). Public trust is important because when the public trusts the health system with their data, the public supports data sharing and storage activities such as the introduction of national electronic health record systems or the build-up of health data cooperatives to pool data for research purposes (Gille and Vayena, 2021). Furthermore, public trust legitimises such health system activities.

To build public trust, we need to understand public trust as an integral part of health policy making and health care activities. Without a sustained focus on and engagement with public trust during the planning, implementation, provision and evaluation phases of health system activities, it is difficult to meaningfully increase and curate public trust. Synthesising from previous work, and encompassing the themes of public trust as presented in Part II of this book, the eight guiding principles in Table 8.1 inform such public trust-building activities (Gille, Smith and Mays, 2022). The guiding principles are aimed at health policy makers and those in charge of steering health system activities, but eventually concern all health system actors that are part of the health system activity where the principles are applied to. The principles should be used collectively and there is no ranking in terms of impact or importance associated to them. In a specific context a ranking would be possible, but the guiding principles as presented in this chapter are aimed at different health system activities in a range of health systems. Even though the underlying evidence was developed from case studies within the public part of the English NHS, I argue that the principles are also useful for other health systems with similar norms and values (Gille, Smith and Mays, 2020). The level of abstraction on the one side allows transferability across different health systems, but on the other side requires that the guiding principles need to be adapted to the context and health system activity in focus.

Table 8.1: Guiding principles to build public trust in health system activities

Do not rush trust building
Engage with the public
Keep the public safe
Offer autonomy to the public
Plan for diverse trust relationships
Recognise that trust is shaped by both emotion and rational thought
Represent the public interest
Work towards realising a net benefit for the health system and the public

Source: Adapted from Gille, Smith and Mays 2022, p 4

1. Do not rush trust building

Building public trust is a commitment to time. Trust does not build under pressure, on the contrary trust grows with patience. We will neither be able to rush trust building, nor should we rush those we trust. A realistic expectation towards the time frame for health policies to unfold their potential to build public trust is important. Unfortunately, little evidence exists that provides an indication of what a realistic time frame is, but slow-growing download rates of tracing apps or vaccination coverage indicate that trust building takes time. We can find similar indications of the time required to build trust in the context of leadership in clinical encounters with women living with HIV; when building trust among stakeholders in environmental sustainability projects; or when building trust in governments more broadly (Blind, 2006; Boschetti et al, 2016; Randolph et al, 2022).

2. Engage with the public

Communication and interaction are the key to trust (Quinn et al, 2013; Yang, Kang and Cha, 2015). Public trust develops from free and open discourse in the public sphere. Health system representatives such as politicians, scientists or health professionals need to firmly engage in public discourse to convey truthful information about the health system activity in focus. Research shows that different health system actors are trusted differently, as politicians are trusted far less to tell the truth as compared to medical staff (Ipsos Mori, 2019). This finding suggests that those health system representatives that are generally more trusted should, where appropriate, be spokespersons of health system activities. That said, all actors responsible for a health care process need to be able to engage with patients and the public in an informed and coordinated way. It is of little use if a politician announces a new health system activity such as the introduction of a health data sharing system, but when a patient asks his/her general practitioner or pharmacist about how the health data will be shared, neither of them have a clue what the patient is talking about.

The trust-building information needs to be understandable, comprehensible and tailored to the public. There is no value in communicating information if the information cannot be understood by the target audience, and if there is no clear purpose of communication. Similarly, being transparent for its own sake is of little use as transparency needs a purpose to be meaningful. The content of communication about a new health system activity should be threefold: Firstly, you want to elicit a feeling of familiarity or comparable positive experiences by relating the new activity to comparable previous health system activities. Here it is important to explain the similarities and differences to help the public to understand better why the new activity is needed and how it differs from the previous. Secondly, you want to explain what the present potential of the health system activity is to achieve the intended benefit. Simply put, if you are not capable of accomplishing in the future what you would like to be trusted for, why should someone trust you? Thirdly, you want to explain what future-facing mechanisms are in place to accomplish the anticipated benefit of the health system activity. There is no doubt that one cannot foresee the future, but you will be able to explain what the expected benefits in the near future are and how you intend to reach the long-term goals in the far future despite increasing uncertainty.

To assess the success of public trust-building engagement and mechanisms, it is crucial to develop evaluation methods; see Chapter Ten. When the results of evaluations uncover problems, or more obvious system scandals occur, open public debate about the issues that led to problems as well as discussions of solutions are necessary to rebuild public trust.

3. Keep the public safe

Patient safety and security in health care are commonly supported features of health systems. The public will not trust a health system with their data if the health system is perceived as unsafe and not capable of keeping health data secure. Therefore, an investment in safety mechanisms and appropriate implementation of legal, behavioural, organisational and technical safeguards is important to gain public trust (Chan et al, 2016).

4. Offer autonomy to the public

Placing trust is a free choice. A classic example of such autonomous choice in health care is the informed consent process where people freely choose to take part in health system activities and where the signature on the consent form can be understood as a sign of trust (Eyal, 2014). Other examples are having control over personal information or opting into a national electronic health record programme. Adhering in practice to the ideal of offering choices to the public and making such choices as a patient is difficult. A range of reasons on patient and system level exist that undermine such choices. A study with patients with psychoses suggests that such patients might feel a threat of coercion, lack information to make choices or lack self-confidence after illness to make a choice. Supportive factors are, for example, time spent with medical staff and knowledge of illness (Laugharne et al, 2012). In the broader context of health care, we might lose autonomy due to our illnesses as we depend on care with the wish for cure. In such situations our choices are often limited, and we do not necessarily perceive them as free choices, especially when treatment options are equally strenuous. On a public policy level, we see that despite the long-lasting push to offer more autonomy to the public, within developed welfare states it is often difficult for members of the public to exercise autonomy due to structural barriers, lack of information and knowledge of alternatives, or lack of equal value alternatives (Burchardt, Evans and Holder, 2015). A challenging discussion in the context of the introduction of national electronic health record systems, tracing apps or organ donation is about whether an opt-in model, where individuals voluntarily take part in such activities, is preferable, or if a default opt-in is desirable where people who do not wish to take part need to opt-out (Moberly, 2014; Morley et al, 2020). Opt-in models need to be citizen-oriented, practical and reasonable. In practice it appears to be challenging to motivate large parts of the public to make such an active opt-in choice. A recent study in the English and Dutch contexts of organ donation provides a positive example from early experiences that moving from an opt-in to an opt-out system is possible with the right levels of public awareness and education, as well as communication strategies in place to gain public support (Jansen et al, 2022). However, in the context of the introduction of national data sharing schemes, the example of the failed care.data initiative in England shows how insufficient communication and lack of public involvement in the design phase of opt-out models contributes in part to the failure of such initiatives due to public perceptions of political paternalism (Carter, Laurie and Dixon-Woods, 2015; Hays and Daker-White, 2015).

These examples illustrate that offering free choice to the public is difficult. Nevertheless, to build trust it is important to provide equal alternatives to those who want to make their own choices, and to equip the public with the knowledge and skills necessary to make free choices. If default opt-in models are in place, it is critical to raise awareness and explain to the public the underlying reasons to gain public trust in the overarching system structure.

5. Plan for diverse trust relationships

The diversity of trust relationships within the concept of public trust in the health system emerges from two trajectories. On the one hand, public trust builds via interactions, experiences and knowledge of a range of different health system actors. For example, we build trust in national electronic health record systems by having a long-lasting relationship with our general practitioner who is a trusted health system representative, and who explains to us the risks and benefits of sharing health data by the means of an electronic health record. At the same time, we saw a convincing interview with a politician and know about the existence of appropriate governance structures and legislation that regulate the access to our data. On the other hand, public trust encompasses a range of other trust concepts, such as self-confidence in our abilities to judge others' trustworthiness, an individual's trust relationship with a health professional or fellow citizen, an individual's trust in a health care institution and the wider system. This draws a complex web of trust relationships (Meyer et al, 2008). This diversity in terms of trust relationships and inherent trust conceptualisations within public trust suggests that a one-size-fits-all approach towards developing public trust-building mechanisms will likely fail. Rather, health policy makers should analyse the context of a given health policy in advance and tailor public trust-building mechanisms in line with the identified trust network.

6. Recognise that trust is shaped by both emotion and rational thought

Most present trust research in health policy and governance suggests that trust establishment is a process of calculated decisions. This synthetic conceptualisation of trust helps to design health policy processes and to build governance processes that mirror trust conceptualisations as they are relatively easy to describe and understand. However, another body of trust research suggests that emotions build trust (Dunn and Schweitzer, 2005; Hartmann, 2015). Sometimes we can articulate and address emotions, such as fear or anger, leading to lower levels of trust. But we also know that at times trusting just feels right, as described by a gut feeling or instinct. The spectrum between calculation and emotion suggests that we need to serve both ends when building public trust.

7. Represent the public interest

Public representation is important to build public trust. If the public perceives politicians or others in public office or those working with public data as a detached elite working for their own interest, the public will lose trust. Guidelines such as the United Kingdom's Nolan Principles of selflessness, integrity, objectivity, accountability, openness, honesty and leadership help to guide government officials towards working in the public interest (Bew, 2015). Despite such guidance, it can be difficult for policy makers and officials to identify what the public interest is. A careful mapping and theorisation of such interests with, for example, citizen engagement exercises can help to define public interest and to guide appropriate behaviour (Tait, 2011).

8. Work towards realising a net benefit for the health system and the public

Public trust develops from a public anticipation of a net benefit resulting from the trusted health care action. The net benefit comprises of four gains: a) an individual benefit; b) a benefit to others; c) a benefit to the health system; and d) a financial benefit to the health system. For example, if health data is used for research, the findings should lead to a net benefit. Private companies working with health data that was donated by patients with altruistic motivations should work towards realising not only a company benefit but also a net benefit. From a public perspective it will be essential that health system actors show their potential, skills and abilities to realise the net benefit they seek to be trusted for.

Concluding remarks

The eight guiding principles to build public trust as a health system actor discussed in this chapter can be used from planning to the evaluation phase of health system activities. Firm engagement in public discourses is imperative to communicate and interact with the public about different health system activities. If those in charge of planning and executing health system activities miss the opportunity to communicate with the public, all further attempts of creating public trust will be challenging. As the health system and living environment is continuously changing, health system actors need to constantly work towards building and maintaining public trust.

NINE

How can we foster public trust by means of effective communications?

It is impossible to establish public trust in the health system without communication, therefore, communication is key to building public trust in the health system. The flow of effective, timely and transparent information is the lifeblood of public trust. Public discourse through online fora, including social media platforms, blogs and media outlets, but also offline in print media and at social gatherings in communal spaces, influence our collective trust in the health system. The diversity of communication platforms allows citizens to simultaneously discuss topical issues with different audiences (see Chapter Four). Key enablers of effective communication in the digital space include: *participation*, where everyone has access to the discourse; *interaction*, where the platform is open to a diverse group of people; *transparency*, where search engines allow users to compile their personalised set of information, and user data allows providers to understand detailed consumer behaviour; *disintermediation*, where journalists are not always necessary anymore to process information and make information publicly available. Today, information sources and consumers can get in direct contact via social media and do not depend as much on traditional media to consolidate and broadcast information (Neuberger, Langenohl and Nuernbergk, 2015; Heinecke, 2019). As search engines foster transparency, companies and their algorithms running search engines play a powerful role in building trust. The overall media has an influential role in shaping trust in medical institutions and public trust more broadly (Mechanic, 1998; Straten, Friele and Groenewegen, 2002).

While social media can be misused to lower public trust by intentionally spreading misinformation, social media is critical for building trust in health policy by enabling transparency and accountability (Limaye et al, 2020). Several media outlets, social media platforms and actors from within and outside the health system navigate in this information space. A 2013 qualitative study with 115 Chinese students using WeChat showed that the type of communication can influence trust. When examining interpersonal, group and mass communication on WeChat, information quality was the only common factor influencing public trust. Other identified trust-building factors were chatting topic, convenience, familiarity, perceived privacy concerns, shared preferences and time saving (Cheng, Fu and de Vreede, 2017, fig 5). Another study conducted in China after the COVID-19 outbreak found that the source credibility, transparency and a reduction in uncertainty build public trust in government policies, as well as in health and political communication (Ngai et al, 2022). A 2009 study with 2,258 participants from the US places an additional emphasis on the opportunity for governments to use social media transparently and thereby build public trust in the government (Song and Lee, 2016). The ability to fulfil promises, good intentions and integrity are key factors influencing trust in consumer health portals that are fora for community exchange in the US (Luo and Najdawi, 2004). The studies make a convincing case for the power of social media discourse to influence levels of public trust in government actions. Factors including transparency, credibility and information quality can contribute to trust building. Intentional social media misuse by spreading misinformation can decrease public trust.

Communication guidelines in the health system context exist to guide public communication strategies. Examples include the World Health Organization (WHO), *WHO outbreak communication planning guide* and *WHO strategic Framework for effective communications* (World Health Organization, 2008, 2017b); the Centers for Disease Control and Prevention (CDC) *Health Communication PLAYBOOK*, the *CDC Clear Communication Index* to aid the development of public communication products, or the CDC *COVID-19 Vaccine Confidence Rapid Community Assessment Guide* (Centers for Disease Control and Prevention, 2018, 2019, 2021); or a range of communication guides issued by the European Centre for Disease Prevention and Control (European Centre for Disease Prevention and Control, 2022). These documents provide structural guidance for different health system actors. Also, most of the guidelines focus on aspects of trust building, but not in detail. Building on the existing guidelines and informed by the work presented in this book, the following ten considerations are designed to guide health system actors in the development of communications that build public trust in the health system:

1. Understand the present and historical context as well as the actors involved in the health system.
2. Understand the mechanisms that are fundamental to building public trust.
3. Understand how public trust-building actions are embedded in the wider societal and political context.
4. Communicate via credible and reputable spokespersons.
5. Make the information easily understandable and tangible, and tailor the information to different target audiences.

6. Convene public discussion fora.
7. Meaningfully engage and involve responsible actors when developing a consistent communication strategy.
8. Provide the opportunity for public engagement and response when developing and implementing communication strategies.
9. Consider the potential impact of conspiracy and misinformation on the public trust-building processes.
10. Develop a contingency plan for events that diminish public trust.

Understand the present and historical context as well as the actors involved in the health system

Precise knowledge about the present and historical context as well as actors involved in the health system is vital. If no full understanding of the context exists, communication strategies are at risk of failing. It is better to acknowledge possible knowledge gaps than pretending to know or inventing knowledge. This book provides an evidence-based conceptual understanding of public trust in the health system that is useful to understand what public trust is and how it develops. It is important to adapt the concept to the applied health system activity and context (Sidani et al, 2010). Careful examination of how public trust unfolds is necessary to understand the cultural and historical particularities of your setting that can influence public trust building. Examples are societal norms and values, collective memories of previous government and health system activities, and the political climate (Gilson, 2003; Papakostas, 2012). In addition to the context, understanding the actors in the health system and how trustful relationships can evolve make it easier to design tailored communication strategies. Public trust is a relational construct in which several actors are involved.

Understand the mechanisms that are fundamental to building public trust

The information communicated to the public should address actions that build public trust: active regulatory systems, anonymity, autonomy, certainty about the future, familiarity, gut feeling, information quality, net benefit, privacy, potential, respect, security and time (Gille, Smith and Mays, 2020). An important question to consider in the development of a communication strategy should be: What activities are in place to adhere to each of the themes? This communication can be categorised along a timeline, with information about the past addressing positive or comparative experiences, as well as the bigger historical context of the health system activity. Information about the present potential to achieve what you ask to be trusted for is crucial. Last, information is needed to explain how the health system activity evolves in the future and how an anticipated net benefit will be achieved. A communication strategy needs to inform about the past, present and future to cover the entire public trust concept.

Understand how public trust-building actions are embedded in the wider societal and political context

A set of framing issues needs to be considered and addressed to show how the health system activity is embedded in the wider societal and political context. These wider issues should not be neglected. Oftentimes when communication strategies and trust-building activities fail, the reason can be found among the issues covered in the framing themes. The issues to consider are reason for the need of public trust; risk; fear; human error (if it occurs); world-views and religion; public mood and zeitgeist; and that trust cannot be expected (Gille, Smith and Mays, 2020). Adequate risk communication is especially important for public trust building. As discussed in the previous chapters, public trust cannot be expected or enforced. It is fundamental to understand that the public assess the trustworthiness of the health system and decides to place trust. Health system actors can assist the process with appropriate communication strategies.

Communicate via credible and reputable spokespersons

The spokespersons of a communication strategy must be perceived by the public as credible and reputable. Common identity cues can further support the trust-building process. In the context of the 2009 H1N1 pandemic in the US, different subpopulations trusted different spokespersons. Therefore, multiple spokespersons targeted to different audiences can be advantageous to trust building, including the opportunity for active engagement with spokespersons on social media (Freimuth et al, 2014).

Make the information easily understandable and tangible, and tailor the information to different target audiences

Communication has little value if we do not understand the information. The information needs to be tailored to the target audience and presented in a format that is easy to understand (Nutbeam, 2000). At the same time it is important to increase public health literacy at community, regional, national and global levels so that the public can follow the information to come to conclusions about trustworthiness (Chen et al, 2018). Shared narratives and publicly relatable user stories can support the trust-building process and exemplify how a health system activity leads to the anticipated success.

Convene public discussion fora

Public trust-building discourse emerges on different communication platforms and physical fora with different population groups and ways of communication. Communication strategies therefore need to operate on different media and social media channels (Snyder, 2007). This is an opportunity to include different spokespersons in the communication strategy to serve the different channels and target audiences.

Meaningfully engage and involve responsible actors when developing a consistent communication strategy

Different health system actors play an important role in the trust-building communication. As a minimum, the actors who engage with patients and members of the public should be able to talk about the health system activity or signpost the patient to an information source. Consistent, timely and transparent communication is important to build public trust (Quinn et al, 2013).

Provide the opportunity for public engagement and response when developing and implementing communication strategies

One-way communication strategies that pour information on the public are not ideal. There should be the option for the public to ask questions and engage in a discourse about a health system activity. Meaningful engagement and involvement at all stages of the communication journey is important. During an active discourse, the necessary information for the trust-building process can be exchanged among members of the public and health system professionals. Essential opportunities are the interactions between patients and health system professionals, but alternative opportunities should also be provided that are outside the care setting. Beyond communication only, engagement of the public in health care planning and health data governance processes builds public trust in such activities (Bruni et al, 2008; Aitken, Cunningham-Burley and Pagliari, 2016). With the ever-changing health system and society, constant engagement with the public will be essential to maintain public trust in digital health intervention and the broader health system (Williams and Fahy, 2019).

Consider the potential impact of conspiracy and misinformation on the public trust-building processes

Conspiracy theories and the intentional spread of misinformation have a negative impact on public trust building. Depending on the health system activity, conspiracy beliefs and misinformation pose considerable competition in the information space and are a threat to a communication strategy. Therefore, a comprehensive understanding of such conspiracy theories and misinformation is required to debunk such theories. People other than medical professionals and politicians are needed to convince conspiracy theorists of the trustworthiness of health system activities (Silver et al, 2022). Therefore, it can be useful to work with influential messengers (Marques, Douglas and Jolley, 2022).

Develop a contingency plan for events that diminish public trust

Unintentional human errors, misconduct, malicious action from external parties and other unexpected events can occur which not only harm the effected, but can scale up to a full-blown media scandal (Blandford, Furniss and Vincent, 2014; Cummings, 2014). Such scandals can lead to reputation loss, financial losses, downfall of public trust and decreasing public acceptance of health system activities. Preparedness and effective crisis management can save image and reputation. 'Crisis response should be well constructed to not leave any room for speculation and possible manipulation by the media in cases of international politics crises. Organisations must explicate the defect in terms that are "believable and cogent" to the public' (Khodarahmi, 2009, p 525). It is naive to assume that such events will not happen in health system activities.

Concluding remarks

Together with existing communication guidelines, the set of ten considerations discussed in this chapter should help to guide health system actors that oversee the design of health communication activities that aim to build public trust.

TEN

How can we foster public trust through effective observation?

Measures of trust and trustworthiness in specific health system activities or the entire health system are useful to monitor and evaluate health system performance (Ozawa and Sripad, 2013; Anderson and Griffith, 2022). We measure 'to provide a reasonable and consistent way to summarize the responses that people make to express their achievements, attitudes, or personal points of view through instruments' (Wilson, 2005, p 5). Declining levels of trust can indicate the need to reform and improve affected health system activities (Abelson, Miller and Giacomini, 2009). Only with a precise understanding of the effect of our actions on levels of public trust can we adapt and revise our actions. Furthermore, evidence about public trust can show if public trust-building mechanisms are cost-effective. The need for accurate trust measurement is highlighted by the Organisation for Economic Co-operation and Development (OECD) and the World Economic Forum (OECD, 2017; World Economic Forum, 2022).

To be able to observe public trust in a meaningful way, we need to have a clear understanding of what public trust is in a specific context (Green and Browne, 2005). As for example presented in the previous chapters of this book, such conceptual precision usually develops from qualitative data, existing literature and detailed research of the concept. If we do not know what we want to measure, we are not able to construct a psychometrically scaled instrument that is valid, reliable and responsive. Any further attempts of measuring are pointless (MacKenzie, 2003). Reliability describes if the measure is free from random error, internally consistent and produces repeatable and unchanging results. Validity describes if the measurement instrument is measuring what it should be measuring. Responsiveness focuses on the ability of the measurement instrument to detect meaningful change over time (Streiner and Norman, 2003; Smith et al, 2005; Gille, 2017, p 28). Trust-specific guidelines and generic guidelines exist to assist the development of a trust-measurement instrument. Following a review of trust measures in health care, Jane Goudge and Lucy Gilson published a best practice research strategy for investigating trust. The strategy follows eight steps (the following is a shortened version, please visit Figure 1, p 1448 in the original reference for detailed guidance) (Goudge and Gilson, 2005, fig 1): 1. Establish rationale for a specific setting; 2. Define research questions; 3. Establish a draft definition; 4. Explore the role and meaning of trust; 5. Examine relationships of trust with other variables; 6. Establish hypotheses; 7.a) Develop a measurement tool and test the tool's validity; 7.b) Use pre-existing questions and data sets; 7.c) Apply experimental studies; 8. Examine the relationship of trust. The first six steps highlight the importance of rigorous groundwork before starting to develop or adapt an existing measure. Another set of guidance are the OECD Guidelines on Measuring Trust. At over 200 pages, the document is a rich and detailed guide covering concept and validity, methodological considerations, trust measurement, and output and data analysis (OECD, 2017). Pointing in the same direction as Goudge and Gilson, the OECD guidelines emphasise that:

In the case of trust, a sound conceptual framework is particularly important. Unlike some relatively straightforward concepts, such as age, gender or marital status, trust is inherently intangible. Although it is possible to observe trusting behaviour and to obtain self-reports from respondents about their stated levels of trust, it is not possible to directly observe trust as such. This raises the issue that respondents might not share a common view of what is meant with respect to trust in a survey question. (OECD, 2017, p 37)

Other useful guidelines exist that explain how measurement instruments should be developed (Lohr, 2002; US Department of Health and Human Services FDA Center for Drug Evaluation and Research, US Department of Health and Human Services FDA Center for Biologics Evaluation and Research, and US Department of Health and Human Services FDA Center for Devices and Radiological Health, 2006; Reeve et al, 2013).

Going back to the 1950s, the landscape of social and political trust measures has evolved since Morris Rosenberg's *Misanthropy and Political Ideology* study (Rosenberg, 1956). Social trust can be loosely defined as a general expectation in other's behaviour (Verducci and Schröer, 2010). Political trust as an indicator for legitimacy can be understood as a general confidence in political institutions (Turper and Aarts, 2017). Three types of trust measures are commonly used: direct trust measures where participants self-report their trust; indirect measures that observe individuals and thereby infer trust; and laboratory experiments that capture behaviour triggered by trust only (Bauer and Freitag, 2017). Academic research and private companies produce large numbers of these different types of measures. A leading systematic review conducted in 2013 by Sachiko Ozawa and Pooja Sripad compared 45 measures of trust in health sector settings. The study revealed that the majority of measures were developed in the United

States of America, half of the measures focus on patient–health care professional relationships, half of the measures were based on qualitative data and 33 per cent were pilot tested (Ozawa and Sripad, 2013). Recent examples of studies measuring levels of public trust include a general population study investigating trust in the health care system and physicians in Croatia. The study used a 90-items questionnaire, of which 49 items were included in the analysis. Findings showed that 58.7 per cent of the respondents displayed high or very high levels of trust in the health care system, 65.6 per cent of the respondents displayed high or very high levels of trust in physicians, and 78.3 per cent of the respondents displayed high or very high levels of trust in a family physician (Nikodem, Ćurković and Borovečki, 2022). A cross-sectional Swedish study using a survey that included a single question on trust showed that 68.5 per cent of respondents had high levels of trust in the health system (Baroudi et al, 2022). In China, the International Social Survey Programme found that 28 per cent of respondents have a great deal or complete trust in China's health system (Zhao, Zhao and Cleary, 2019). In 2002, Straten, Friele and Groenewegen developed a public trust in the Dutch health care system measure (Straten, Friele and Groenewegen, 2002). Afterwards, the measure was used for example in a comparative study in Germany, the Netherlands, England and Wales as well as adapted for Trinidad and Tobago (Schee et al, 2007; Peters and Youssef, 2016). With 37 items, the instrument covers six dimensions of public trust: patient focus of providers; policies at the macro level be without consequences for the patient; health care providers' expertise; quality of care; information supply and communication by care providers; and quality of cooperation (Straten, Friele and Groenewegen, 2002, p 231). Straten and colleagues understood that:

Public trust in health care could be defined as being confident that you will be adequately treated when you are in need of health care. … Public trust can be seen as a generalized attitude based on personal experience in trust situations, on direct communication of other people's experience and on mass media communication. In its turn, public trust influences the way individuals react in interpersonal trust situations. (Straten, Friele and Groenewegen, 2002, pp 227–8)

Outside of health system research, the Global Trust Inventory (building on the World Values Survey) consists of 24 items to collect data about trust in domestic, international, governmental and non-governmental institutions (Liu et al, 2018). Other, well-known examples of trust and public trust measurement activities are the Edelman Trust Barometer, conducted by the global communication firm Edelman (Daniel J. Edelman Holdings, Inc.) with a 2022 special report on trust and health stating that trust is a key determinant of health; different trust measurement studies conducted by the international market and social research company Ipsos; international trust in government studies conducted by the OECD; questions about trust being part of the Eurobarometer collecting European public opinion data commissioned by the European Commission, the European Parliament and further EU institutions and agencies; and, questions about trust as part of the European Social Survey conducted by the European Social Survey European Research Infrastructure Consortium (Daniel J. Edelman Holdings, Inc., 2022b, 2022a; European Parliament, 2022; Ipsos, 2022; OECD, 2022; The European Social Survey European Research Infrastructure Consortium, 2022).

The variety of measurement instruments show a wide range of different forms of asking participants about trust. Some mirror themes of an underlying conceptual framework of trust, others ask directly in how far participants trust X. This pot-pourri makes comparison between studies difficult. When comparing studies with a similar focus we also miss comparability due to different underlying conceptualisations of trust (Gille, 2017, chapter 3). As trust is context specific, this mix of measures is not necessarily surprising because we need tailored approaches to trust measurement that fits the research context. However, for reasons of comparability, it would be beneficial to use commonly accepted measures of public trust in the health system. Building on the trust measurement guidelines and the conceptual framework presented in this book, I suggest developing a comprehensive measurement instrument where the questions emerge from the conceptual themes. Asking only questions about the effect of public trust, participation and legitimacy is in my view of little use for policy making, as we will have no indication of why participation levels go down or rise if we only know that participation levels change. We want to understand why this is the case and what we need to adjust in our policy or actions, see Figure 10.1.

Unquestionably, it is reasonable to also collect data about the effects of public trust such as, for example, download rates of medical apps, but we cannot derive much meaningful information from those numbers if we aim to inform health policy making. Eventually, in many cases we will not even know with exactitude if participation rates increase or decrease

Figure 10.1: Schematic link of conceptual themes – governance and policy actions – measurement questions

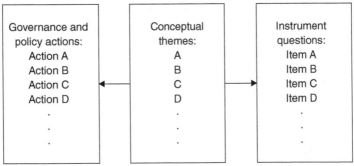

because of changing levels of public trust as public trust is by no means the only cause for participation and legitimacy. We might use a medical app, because if we do not use the app we will not have full access to care. Or we download a COVID-19 contact tracing app because a restaurant only permits access if you have an active contact tracing app. Both cases have little to do with trust.

Asking participants directly about trust by using the word trust in the questions is a way of constructing an instrument that might initially seem intuitive. We could simply ask 'Do you trust the health system with your data?' and the response options could be a simple binary 'yes' and 'no' answer or a Likert type (Duncan and Stenbeck, 1987; Harpe, 2015). The answer to such a question produces information about the percentage of participants trusting the health system to what degree. Such information can be useful to understand proportions of society and, for example, analysed in correlation with respondents' postcodes we can then map in which region people seem to trust more or trust less. Yet, again, this information is only of limited use if we want to understand what we need to do to increase levels of trust.

In contrast, we can develop a comprehensive measurement instrument (Wilson, 2005, p 27). This way we receive a detailed picture of which areas of the public trust-building process works well and which areas need adjustment. For example, if the responses show that respondents find data privacy troublesome, we know that we need to adjust our data privacy policy. The same counts for all other themes.

Concluding remarks

To conclude, a wide array of trust and public trust measurement instruments for a diverse range of health system contexts exist. The many instruments led to a hodge-podge of ways to measure trust which makes comparison of results difficult.

Considering the wish to inform health policy making and governance with an instrument to quantify public trust, such an instrument should be constructed based on comprehensive conceptualisation of public trust.

ELEVEN

Conclusion

This book provides an evidence and theory-based explanation of public trust in the health system with the aim to inform health policy making, health system governance and health professionals' actions. The example of health data use in health care shows that public trust is pivotal for the success of health system activities and that public trust should be considered as an integral component for policies.

As Luhmann already indicated in the 1970s, and what remains true in the future, with the increasing technologisation of societies and systems, trust will become increasingly important (Luhmann, 2017). In its capacity to simplify the world around us and thereby reduce complexity, trust empowers us to act and partake in complex activities such as health system activities. We witnessed in recent years a series of system shake-ups that introduced uncertainty into, for many of us, perceived stable living environments, societal systems and state structures. From a European perspective some examples are the 2015 Syrian refugee crisis, the rise of right-wing populism across Europe, the COVID-19 pandemic, and the 2020 Brexit. With a future-facing view, many anticipate that climate change will lead to further global public health challenges and social uncertainties. With the advancement of digital health, the international movement of people and the wish for smooth health data transfers between health care actors both nationally and internationally, public trust in such health data use will remain an important topic in the coming years. I hypothesise that such developments and impacts on society led to the surfacing of trust in public debate and consequently for many of us the perceived importance of trust. As public trust has the capacity to build social cohesion and to contribute to stable, safe and prosperous societies, we will need to continue our efforts to build public trust where necessary and protect high levels of public trust where possible. In response to this need, and building on the previous chapters, I raise several questions that need to be answered by future research and health system actions:

How can we evaluate the performance of health policies to build public trust?

When we design health policies with the intention to increase public trust in a specific health system activity, we need to be able to evaluate if such health policies meet their target. Only if we have a precise understanding of the problems in terms of public trust building will we be able to adjust health policies and health care activities. To do so, it will not be sufficient to monitor the possible effects of public trust such as download rates of medical apps or vaccination rates. Rather, we will also need to monitor the actions that build trust, such as, for example, adherence to legislation, privacy protection or the enablement of public choices; see Chapter Five. We should develop ways that assess all conceptual themes of public trust to understand public issues emerging around such themes. This way we can confront rising problems with meaningful policy interventions and health system actions.

What is the economic power of public trust in health systems?

We know from our daily life and research that trust is of extreme value for the economy. A considerable amount of behavioural economics research emerged around trust (Berg, Dickhaut and McCabe, 1995; Johnson and Mislin, 2011) as well as research about the financial impact of reputation losses of companies due to different reasons (reputation may be understand as a synonym or part of trustworthiness) (Garg, Curtis and Halper, 2003; Gatzert, 2015). Throughout recent years, I witnessed at several conferences that private companies in health care talk about the importance of maintaining high levels of trust in their products and therefore the need to invest resources in trust-building mechanisms. Consumer trust is understood to be critical for sales and consumer satisfaction. If trust is lost, we can look at legal costs, drops in company share values, loss of employees, increase of transaction costs, decrease of sales or failure altogether. The costs of misplaced trust as well as misused trust could have a significant effect for health system actors and the public. Yet with a more positive view, we do not find many studies that look at costs saved due to increased levels of trust or investigating the financial return gained by trust-building mechanisms.

How does public trust develop in unstable societies?

Most of trust research emerged and still emerges in Europe and the United States of America (Ozawa and Sripad, 2013). When considering conflicts around the globe and their impact on health systems and the delivery of care, we need to understand how public trust can be built in unstable societies and within peace negotiations (Told, 2022).

How does public trust develop in international and national health politics?

With the introduction of the European Health Data Space and in the context of globalisation, international health data transfer and data use will continue to grow. Global public health threats such as pandemics or climate change require globally coordinated health policies. To adhere to such policies, public trust not only needs to develop in national political structures but also in international political authorities and foreign institutions. We need research to support these trust-establishment processes with evidence.

How does history influence trust in present digital health activities?

Numerous studies provide evidence for the strong effect of history and collective memory on present trust building in health system activities. When we think about artificial intelligence, pan-European electronic health systems or other modern health system activities, we tend to overlook potential links to historic health system activities. When designing digital health activities, we need to understand what experiences exist within societies that can influence the public participation process in such activities.

While reading this introductory book, I hope you identified many more areas of future action or open questions that need to be addressed to build public trust. With constantly changing health systems and societies, we will need to continuously refine our understanding of public trust to be able to build public trust where needed.

References

Abelson, J., Miller, F.A. and Giacomini, M. (2009) 'What does it mean to trust a health system? A qualitative study of Canadian health care values', *Health Policy*, 91(1), pp 63–70. https://doi.org/10.1016/j.healthpol.2008.11.006

Abouelmehdi, K., Beni-Hessane, A. and Khaloufi, H. (2018) 'Big healthcare data: preserving security and privacy', *Journal of Big Data*, 5(1), p 1. https://doi.org/10.1186/s40537-017-0110-7

Adjekum, A., Blasimme, A. and Vayena, F. (2018) 'Elements of trust in digital health systems: scoping review', *J Med Internet Res*, 20(12), p e11254. https://doi.org/10.2196/11254

Ahorsu, D.K. et al (2022) 'The mediational role of trust in the healthcare system in the association between generalized trust and willingness to get COVID-19 vaccination in Iran', *Human Vaccines & Immunotherapeutics*, 18(1), pp 1–8. https://doi.org/10.1080/21645515.2021.1993689

Aitken, M., Cunningham-Burley, S. and Pagliari, C. (2016) 'Moving from trust to trustworthiness: experiences of public engagement in the Scottish Health Informatics Programme', *Science and Public Policy*, 43(5), pp 713–23. https://doi.org/10.1093/scipol/scv075

Alhaffar, M.H.D.B.A. and Janos, S. (2021) 'Public health consequences after ten years of the Syrian crisis: a literature review', *Globalization and Health*, 17(111), pp 1–11. https://doi.org/10.1186/s12992-021-00762-9

Altomonte, C. and Villafranca, A. (eds) (2019) *Europe in Identity Crisis. The Future of the EU in the Age of Nationalism*. Milan: Ledizioni. https://doi.org/10.14672/55261579

Anderson, A. and Griffith, D.M. (2022) 'Measuring the trustworthiness of health care organizations and systems', *The Milbank Quarterly*, 100(2), pp 345–64. https://doi.org/10.1111/1468-0009.12564

Andrade, G. (2020) 'Medical conspiracy theories: cognitive science and implications for ethics', *Medicine, Health Care and Philosophy*, 23(3), pp 505–18. https://doi.org/10.1007/s11019-020-09951-6

Apeti, A.E. (2022) 'Does trust in government improve Covid-19's crisis management?', *SN Social Sciences*, 2(202), pp 1–21. Ahttps://doi.org/10.1007/s43545-022-00505-6

Asensio, M. (2021) 'The political legitimacy of the healthcare system in Portugal: insights from the European Social Survey', *Healthcare*, 9(2), p 202. https://doi.org/10.3390/healthcare9020202

Bacharach, M. and Gambetta, D. (2001) 'Trust in signs', in K.S. Cook (ed) *Trust in Society*, Russell Sage Foundation, pp 148–84. Available from: http://www.jstor.org/stable/10.7758/978161 0441322.9 (Accessed: 24 April 2022).

Baier, D. and Manzoni, P. (2020) 'Verschwörungsmentalität und Extremismus – Befunde aus Befragungsstudien in der Schweiz', *Monatsschrift für Kriminologie und Strafrechtsreform*, 103(2), pp 83–96. https://doi.org/10.1515/mks-2020-2044

Banner, N. (2022) 'NHS data breaches: a further erosion of trust', *BMJ*, 377, p o1187. https://doi.org/10.1136/bmj.o1187

Baroudi, M. et al (2022) 'Social factors associated with trust in the health system in northern Sweden: a cross-sectional study', *BMC Public Health*, 22(1), p 881. https://doi.org/10.1186/s12 889-022-13332-4

Bates, D.W. et al (1999) 'The impact of computerized physician order entry on medication error prevention', *Journal of the American Medical Informatics Association*, 6(4), pp 313–21. https://doi.org/10.1136/jamia.1999.00660313

Bauer, P.C. and Freitag, M. (2017) 'Measuring trust', in E.M. Uslaner (ed) *The Oxford Handbook of Social and Political Trust*, Oxford University Press, pp 15–36. https://doi.org/10.1093/oxfordhb/9780190274801.013.1

Baum, N.M., Jacobson, P.D. and Goold, S.D. (2009) '"Listen to the people": public deliberation about social distancing measures in a pandemic', *The American Journal of Bioethics*, 9(11), pp 4–14. https://doi.org/10.1080/15265160903197531

Bekker, M., Ivankovic, D. and Biermann, O. (2020) 'Early lessons from COVID-19 response and shifts in authority: public trust, policy legitimacy and political inclusion', *European Journal of Public Health*, 30(5), pp 854–5. https://doi.org/10.1093/eurpub/ckaa181

Belfrage, S., Helgesson, G. and Lynøe, N. (2022) 'Trust and digital privacy in healthcare: a cross-sectional descriptive study of trust and attitudes towards uses of electronic health data among the general public in Sweden', *BMC Medical Ethics*, 23: 19. https://doi.org/10.1186/s12910-022-00758-z

Bellatin, A. et al (2021) 'Overcoming vaccine deployment challenges among the hardest to reach: lessons from polio elimination in India', *BMJ Global Health*, 6(4), p e005125. https://doi.org/10.1136/bmjgh-2021-005125

Bellazzi, F. and Boyneburgk, K.V. (2020) 'COVID-19 calls for virtue ethics', *Journal of Law and the Biosciences*, 7(1), p lsaa056. https://doi.org/10.1093/jlb/lsaa056

Benjamins, M.R. (2006) 'Religious influences on trust in physicians and the health care aystem', *The International Journal of Psychiatry in Medicine*, 36(1), pp 69–83. https://doi.org/10.2190/EKJ2-BCCT-8LT4-K01W

Berg, J., Dickhaut, J. and McCabe, K. (1995) 'Trust, reciprocity, and social history', *Games and Economic Behavior*, 10(1), pp 122–42. https://doi.org/10.1006/game.1995.1027

Bergman, B., Neuhauser, D. and Provost, L. (2011) 'Five main processes in healthcare: a Citizen Perspective', *BMJ Quality & Safety*, 20(Suppl 1), p i41. https://doi.org/10.1136/bmjqs.2010.046409

Bew, P. (2015) 'The Committee on Standards in Public Life: twenty years of the Nolan Principles 1995–2015', *The Political Quarterly*, 86(3), pp 411–18. https://doi.org/10.1111/1467-923X.12176

Bjørnskov, C. (2007) 'Determinants of generalized trust: a cross-country comparison', *Public Choice*, 130(1–2), pp 1–21. https://doi.org/10.1007/s11127-006-9069-1

Blair, R.A., Morse, B.S. and Tsai, L.L. (2017) 'Public health and public trust: survey evidence from the Ebola virus disease epidemic in Liberia', *Social Science & Medicine*, 172, pp 89–97. https://doi.org/10.1016/j.socscimed.2016.11.016

Blandford, A., Furniss, D. and Vincent, C. (2014) 'Patient safety and interactive medical devices: realigning work as imagined and work as done', *Clinical Risk*, 20(5), pp 107–10. https://doi.org/10.1177/1356262214556550

Blasimme, A. and Vayena, E. (2020) 'What's next for COVID-19 apps? Governance and oversight', *Science*, 370(6518), pp 760–2. https://doi.org/10.1126/science.abd9006

Bleetman, A. et al (2012) 'Human factors and error prevention in emergency medicine', *Emergency Medicine Journal*, 29(5), pp 389–93. https://doi.org/10.1136/emj.2010.107698

Blind, P.K. (2006) *Building Trust in Government in the Twenty-First Century: Review of Literature and Emerging Issues*. New York: United Nations Department of Economic and Social Affairs, p 31.

Bogart, L.M. et al (2010) 'Conspiracy beliefs about HIV are related to antiretroviral treatment nonadherence among African American men with HIV', *JAIDS Journal of Acquired Immune Deficiency Syndromes*, 53(5), pp 648–55. https://doi.org/10.1097/QAI.0b013e3181c57dbc

Bogart, L.M. and Thorburn, S. (2005) 'Are HIV/AIDS conspiracy beliefs a barrier to HIV prevention among African Americans?', *JAIDS Journal of Acquired Immune Deficiency Syndromes*, 38(2), pp 213–18. Available from: https://journals.lww.com/jaids/Fulltext/2005/02010/Are_HIV_AIDS_Conspiracy_Beliefs_a_Barrier_to_HIV.14.aspx (Accessed: 12 July 2023).

Bohnet, I. and Zeckhauser, R. (2004) 'Trust, risk and betrayal', *Trust and Trustworthiness*, 55(4), pp 467–84. https://doi.org/10.1016/j.jebo.2003.11.004

Borah, P., Irom, B. and Hsu, Y.C. (2021) '"It infuriates me": examining young adults' reactions to and recommendations to fight misinformation about COVID-19', *Journal of Youth Studies*, 25(10), pp 1–21. https://doi.org/10.1080/13676261.2021.1965108

Boschetti, F. et al (2016) 'A call for empirically based guidelines for building trust among stakeholders in environmental sustainability projects', *Sustainability Science*, 11(5), pp 855–9. https://doi.org/10.1007/s11625-016-0382-4

Boufides, C.H., Gable, L. and Jacobson, P.D. (2019) 'Learning from the Flint water crisis: restoring and improving public health practice, accountability, and trust', *The Journal of Law, Medicine & Ethics*, 47(Suppl 2), pp 23–6. https://doi.org/10.1177/1073110519857310

Branzei, O., Vertinsky, I. and Camp, R.D. (2007) 'Culture-contingent signs of trust in emergent relationships', *Organizational Behavior and Human Decision Processes*, 104(1), pp 61–82. https://doi.org/10.1016/j.obhdp.2006.11.002

Braun, D. and Trüdinger, E.-M. (2022) 'Communal and exchange-based trust in Germany thirty years after reunification: convergence or still an East–West divide?', *German Politics*, 32(1), pp 43–62. https://doi.org/10.1080/09644008.2022.2054989

Briggs, C.L. (2004) 'Theorizing modernity conspiratorially: science, scale, and the political economy of public discourse in explanations of a cholera epidemic', *American Ethnologist*, 31(2), pp 164–87. https://doi.org/10.1525/ae.2004.31.2.164

Brotherton, R., French, C.C. and Pickering, A.D. (2013) 'Measuring belief in conspiracy theories: the generic conspiracist beliefs scale', *Frontiers in Psychology*, 4, p 279. https://doi.org/10.3389/fpsyg.2013.00279

Bruder, M. and Kunert, L. (2021) 'The conspiracy hoax? Testing key hypotheses about the correlates of generic beliefs in conspiracy theories during the COVID-19 pandemic', *International Journal of Psychology*, 57(1), pp 43–8. https://doi.org/10.1002/ijop.12769

Bruni, R.A. et al (2008) 'Public engagement in setting priorities in health care', *Canadian Medical Association Journal*, 179(1), pp 15–18. https://doi.org/10.1503/cmaj.071656

Burchardt, T., Evans, M. and Holder, H. (2015) 'Public policy and inequalities of choice and autonomy', *Social Policy & Administration*, 49(1), pp 44–67. https://doi.org/10.1111/spol.12074

Butt, S.A. et al (2022) 'A multivariant secure framework for smart mobile health application', Transactions on Emerging Telecommunications Technologies, 33(8). https://doi.org/10.1002/ett.3684

Cairney, P. and Wellstead, A. (2020) 'COVID-19: effective policymaking depends on trust in experts, politicians, and the public', *Policy Design and Practice*, 4(1), pp 1–14. https://doi.org/10.1080/25741292.2020.1837466

Calnan, M. and Rowe, R. (2008) *Trust Matters in Health Care*. Maidenhead: Open University Press.

Carter, P., Laurie, G.T. and Dixon-Woods, M. (2015) 'The social licence for research: why care.data ran into trouble', *Journal of Medical Ethics*, 41(5), pp 404–9. https://doi.org/10.1136/medethics-2014-102374

Celum, C. et al (2020) 'Covid-19, Ebola, and HIV – leveraging lessons to maximize impact', *New England Journal of Medicine*, 383(19), p e106. https://doi.org/10.1056/NEJMp2022269

Centers for Disease Control and Prevention (2018) *Health Communication PLAYBOOK*. Available from: https://www.cdc.gov/nceh/clearwriting/docs/health-comm-playbook-508.pdf (Accessed: 20 October 2022).

Centers for Disease Control and Prevention (2019) *CDC Clear Communication Index*. Available from: https://www.cdc.gov/ccindex/pdf/clear-communication-user-guide.pdf (Accessed: 21 October 2022).

Centers for Disease Control and Prevention (2021) *COVID-19 Vaccine Confidence Rapid Community Assessment Guide*. Available from: https://www.cdc.gov/vaccines/covid-19/vaccinate-with-confidence/rca-guide/downloads/CDC-RCA-Guide-2021-508.pdf (Accessed: 21 October 2022).

Chambers, S. (2021) 'Truth, deliberative democracy, and the virtues of accuracy: is fake news destroying the public sphere?', *Political Studies*, 69(1), pp 147–63. https://doi.org/10.1177/0032321719890811

Chan, T. et al (2016) 'UK National Data Guardian for health and care's review of data security: trust, better security and opt-outs', *BMJ Health & Care Informatics*, 23(3), pp 627–32. https://doi.org/10.14236/jhi.v23i3.909

Chen, X. et al (2018) 'Health literacy and use and trust in health information', *Journal of Health Communication*, 23(8), pp 724–34. https://doi.org/10.1080/10810730.2018.1511658

Cheng, X., Fu, S. and de Vreede, G.-J. (2017) 'Understanding trust influencing factors in social media communication: a qualitative study', *International Journal of Information Management*, 37(2), pp 25–35. https://doi.org/10.1016/j.ijinfomgt.2016.11.009

Cheung, A.H.S., Alden, D.L. and Wheeler, M.S. (1998) 'Cultural attitudes of Asian-Americans toward death adversely impact organ donation', *Transplantation Proceedings*, 30(7), pp 3609–10. https://doi.org/10.1016/S0041-1345(98)01156-7

Chu, J., Pink, S.L. and Willer, R. (2021) 'Religious identity cues increase vaccination intentions and trust in medical experts among American Christians', *Proceedings of the National Academy of Sciences*, 118(49), p e2106481118. https://doi.org/10.1073/pnas.2106481118

Coventry, L. and Branley, D. (2018) 'Cybersecurity in healthcare: a narrative review of trends, threats and ways forward', *Maturitas*, 113, pp 48–52. https://doi.org/10.1016/j.maturitas.2018.04.008

Cummings, L. (2014) 'The "trust" heuristic: arguments from authority in public health', *Health Communication*, 29(10), pp 1043–56. https://doi.org/10.1080/10410236.2013.831685

Damschroder, L.J. et al (2007) 'Patients, privacy and trust: patients' willingness to allow researchers to access their medical records', *Social Science and Medicine*, 64(1), pp 223–35. https://doi.org/10.1016/j.socscimed.2006.08.045

Dane, E., Rockmann, K.W. and Pratt, M.G. (2012) 'When should I trust my gut? Linking domain expertise to intuitive decision-making effectiveness', *Organizational Behavior and Human Decision Processes*, 119(2), pp 187–94. https://doi.org/10.1016/j.obhdp.2012.07.009

Daniel J. Edelman Holdings, Inc. (2022a) '2022 Edelman Trust Barometer Special Report: Trust and Health'. Available from: https://www.edelman.com/trust/22/special-report-trust-in-health (Accessed: 13 October 2022).

Daniel J. Edelman Holdings, Inc. (2022b) 'Why we study trust'. Available from: https://www.edelman.com/trust (Accessed: 12 October 2022).

Degerli, M. (2023) 'Privacy issues in data-driven health care', in N. Dey (ed) *Data-Driven Approach for Bio-medical and Healthcare*, Singapore: Springer Nature Singapore, pp 23–37. https://doi.org/10.1007/978-981-19-5184-8_2

Dellmuth, L. et al (2022) *Citizens, Elites, and the Legitimacy of Global Governance*, Oxford: Oxford University Press. https://doi.org/10.1093/oso/9780192856241.001.0001

Deml, M.J. et al (2019) 'Determinants of vaccine hesitancy in Switzerland: study protocol of a mixed-methods national research programme', *BMJ Open*, 9(11), p e032218. https://doi.org/10.1136/bmjopen-2019-032218

Deschênes, M. and Sallée, C. (2005) 'Accountability in population biobanking: comparative approaches', *The Journal of Law, Medicine & Ethics*, 33(1), pp 40–53. https://doi.org/10.1111/j.1748-720X.2005.tb00209.x

Deurenberg-Yap, M. et al (2005) 'The Singaporean response to the SARS outbreak: knowledge sufficiency versus public trust', *Health Promotion International*, 20(4), pp 320–6. https://doi.org/10.1093/heapro/dai010

Deutscher Paritätischer Wohlfahrtsverband, Landesverband Berlin e.V. (2022) 'Heil- und Pflegeanstalt Hall in Tirol (Landeskrankenhaus Hall)'. Available from: https://www.gedenkort-t4.eu/historische-orte/heil-und-pflegeanstalt-hall-in-tirol-landeskrankenhaus-hall (Accessed: 12 October 2022).

Devine, D. et al (2021) 'Trust and the Coronavirus pandemic: what are the consequences of and for trust? An early review of the literature', *Political Studies Review*, 19(2), pp 274–85. https://doi.org/10.1177/1478929920948684

van Dijck, J. and Alinejad, D. (2020) 'Social media and trust in scientific expertise: debating the Covid-19 pandemic in the Netherlands', *Social Media + Society*, 6(4), p 2056305120981057. https://doi.org/10.1177/2056305120981057

Dohle, S., Wingen, T. and Schreiber, M. (2020) 'Acceptance and adoption of protective measures during the COVID-19 pandemic: the role of trust in politics and trust in science', *Social Psychological Bulletin*, 15(4), p e4315. https://doi.org/10.32872/spb.4315

Douglas, K.M. et al (2019) 'Understanding conspiracy theories', *Political Psychology*, 40(S1), pp 3–35. https://doi.org/10.1111/pops.12568

Duncan, G. (2007) 'Privacy by design', *Science*, 317(5842), pp 1178–9. https://doi.org/10.1126/science.1143464

Duncan, O.D. and Stenbeck, M. (1987) 'Are Likert scales unidimensional?', *Social Science Research*, 16(3), pp 245–59. https://doi.org/10.1016/0049-089X(87)90003-2

Dunn, J.R. and Schweitzer, M.E. (2005) 'Feeling and believing: the influence of emotion on trust', *Journal of Personality and Social Psychology*, 88(5), pp 736–48. https://doi.org/10.1037/0022-3514.88.5.736

Earle, T.C. (2010) 'Trust in risk management: a model-based review of empirical research', *Risk Analysis*, 30(4), pp 541–74. https://doi.org/10.1111/j.1539-6924.2010.01398.x

Earle, T. and Siegrist, M. (2008) 'Trust, confidence and cooperation model: a framework for understanding the relation between trust and risk perception', *International Journal of Global Environmental Issues*, 8(1/2), pp 17–29. https://doi.org/10.1504/IJGENVI.2008.017257

Einstein, A. (1954) *Ideas and Opinions*. New York: Crown.

Elena-Bucea, A. et al (2021) 'Assessing the role of age, education, gender and income on the digital divide: evidence for the European Union', *Information Systems Frontiers*, 23(4), pp 1007–21. https://doi.org/10.1007/s10796-020-10012-9

Elo, S. and Kyngäs, H. (2008) 'The qualitative content analysis process', *Journal of Advanced Nursing*, 62(1), pp 107–15. https://doi.org/10.1111/j.1365-2648.2007.04569.x

Engdahl, E. and Lidskog, R. (2014) 'Risk, communication and trust: towards an emotional understanding of trust', *Public Understanding of Science*, 23(6), pp 703–17. https://doi.org/10.1177/096366251 2460953

Entwistle, V.A. and Quick, O. (2006) 'Trust in the context of patient safety problems', *Journal of Health Organization and Management*, 20(5), pp 397–416. https://doi.org/10.1108/1477726061 0701786

Erikson, E.H. (1950) *Childhood and Society*. New York, NY: Norton.

European Centre for Disease Prevention and Control (2017) *Catalogue of Interventions Addressing Vaccine Hesitancy*. Stockholm: ECDC. https://data.europa.eu/doi/10.2900/654210 (Accessed: 17 June 2022).

European Centre for Disease Prevention and Control (2022) *Communication Guides, European Centre for Disease Prevention and Control*. Available from: https://www.ecdc.europa.eu/en/hea lth-communication/communication-reports/guides (Accessed: 1 November 2022).

European Commission (2022a) *2022 Strengthened Code of Practice on Disinformation*. Available from: https://digital-strategy.ec.europa. eu/en/library/2022-strengthened-code-practice-disinformation (Accessed: 12 January 2023).

European Commission (2022b) *Signatories of the 2022 Strengthened Code of Practice on Disinformation*. Available from: https://digi tal-strategy.ec.europa.eu/en/library/signatories-2022-strengthe ned-code-practice-disinformation (Accessed: 12 January 2023).

European Observatory on Health Systems and Policies, Fahy, N. and Williams, G.A. (2021) *Use of digital health tools in Europe: before, during and after COVID-19*, Copenhagen: World Health Organization. Regional Office for Europe (Health Systems and Policy Analysis; 42). Available from: https://apps.who.int/iris/ handle/10665/345091 (Accessed: 12 July 2023).

European Parliament (2022) 'Eurobarometer'. Available from: https://www.europarl.europa.eu/at-your-service/en/be-heard/euroba rometer (Accessed: 12 October 2022).

Eyal, N. (2014) 'Using informed consent to save trust', *Journal of Medical Ethics*, 40(7), pp 437–44. https://doi.org/10.1136/medeth ics-2012-100490

Fang, W. et al (2017) 'A survey of big data security and privacy preserving', *IETE Technical Review*, 34(5), pp 544–60. https://doi.org/10.1080/02564602.2016.1215269

Farrar, J.J. and Piot, P. (2014) 'The Ebola emergency – immediate action, ongoing strategy', *New England Journal of Medicine*, 371(16), pp 1545–6. https://doi.org/10.1056/NEJMe1411471

Ferrario, A., Loi, M. and Viganò, E. (2020) 'In AI we trust incrementally: a multi-layer model of trust to analyze human-artificial intelligence interactions', *Philosophy & Technology*, 33(3), pp 523–39. https://doi.org/10.1007/s13347-019-00378-3

Ferrera, M.J. et al (2016) 'Embedded mistrust then and now: findings of a focus group study on African American perspectives on breast cancer and its treatment', *Critical Public Health*, 26(4), pp 455–65. https://doi.org/10.1080/09581596.2015.1117576

de Figueiredo, A. et al (2020) 'Mapping global trends in vaccine confidence and investigating barriers to vaccine uptake: a large-scale retrospective temporal modelling study', *The Lancet*, 396(10255), pp 898–908. https://doi.org/10.1016/S0140-6736(20)31558-0

Foley, K. et al (2021) 'Exploring access to, use of and benefits from population-oriented digital health services in Australia', *Health Promotion International*, 36(4), pp 1105–15. https://doi.org/10.1093/heapro/daaa145

Ford, E. et al (2019) 'Our data, our society, our health: a vision for inclusive and transparent health data science in the United Kingdom and beyond', *Learning Health Systems*, 3(3), p e10191. https://doi.org/10.1002/lrh2.10191

Freeman, D. et al (2020) 'Coronavirus conspiracy beliefs, mistrust, and compliance with government guidelines in England', *Psychological Medicine*, 52(2), pp 251–63. https://doi.org/10.1017/S00332 91720001890

Freimuth, V.S. et al (2014) 'Trust during the early stages of the 2009 H1N1 pandemic', *Journal of Health Communication*, 19(3), pp 321–39. https://doi.org/10.1080/10810730.2013.811323

Frevert, U. (2013) *Vertrauensfragen: eine Obsession der Moderne*, Originalau. München: Beck.

Fukuyama, F. (1995) *Trust: The Social Virtues and the Creation of Prosperity*, New York, NY: Free Press.

Gambetta, D. (2011) 'Signaling', in P. Bearman and P. Hedström (eds) *The Oxford Handbook of Analytical Sociology*, Oxford University Press, pp 168–94. https://doi.org/10.1093/oxfordhb/978019 9215362.013.8

Garg, A., Curtis, J. and Halper, H. (2003) 'Quantifying the financial impact of IT security breaches', *Information Management & Computer Security*, 11(2), pp 74–83. https://doi.org/10.1108/09685220310468646

Gasser, U. et al (2020) 'Digital tools against COVID-19: taxonomy, ethical challenges, and navigation aid', *The Lancet Digital Health*, 2(8), pp e425–e434. https://doi.org/10.1016/S2589-7500(20)30137-0

Gatzert, N. (2015) 'The impact of corporate reputation and reputation damaging events on financial performance: empirical evidence from the literature', *European Management Journal*, 33(6), pp 485–99. https://doi.org/10.1016/j.emj.2015.10.001

Gehman, J., Lefsrud, L.M. and Fast, S. (2017) 'Social license to operate: legitimacy by another name?', *Canadian Public Administration*, 60(2), pp 293–317. https://doi.org/10.1111/capa.12218

Geisler, A.M. (2022) 'Public trust in citizens' juries when the people decide on policies: evidence from Switzerland', *Policy Studies*, pp 1–20. https://doi.org/10.1080/01442872.2022.2091125

Genomics England (2022) *100,000 Genomes Project*, [online]. Available from: https://www.genomicsengland.co.uk/initiatives/100000-genomes-project (Accessed: 22 October 2022).

Ghafur, S. et al (2020) 'Public perceptions on data sharing: key insights from the UK and the USA', *The Lancet Digital Health*, 2(9), pp e444–e446. https://doi.org/10.1016/S2589-7500(20)30161-8

Giddens, A. (1990) *The Consequences of Modernity*, Cambridge: Polity Press.

Gille, F. (2017) *Theory and conceptualisation of public trust in the health care system: Three English case studies: care.data, biobanks and 100,000 Genomes Project,* PhD thesis, London School of Hygiene & Tropical Medicine. https://doi.org/10.17037/PUBS.04645534

Gille, F. (2022) 'About the essence of trust: tell the truth and let me choose – I might trust you', *International Journal of Public Health*, 67. https://doi.org/10.3389/ijph.2022.1604592

Gille, F. and Brall, C. (2020) 'Public trust: caught between hype and need', *International Journal of Public Health*, 65, pp 233–4. https://doi.org/10.1007/s00038-020-01343-0

Gille, F. and Brall, C. (2021a) 'Can we know if donor trust expires? About trust relationships and time in the context of open consent for future data use', *Journal of Medical Ethics*, 48(3), pp 184–8. https://doi.org/10.1136/medethics-2020-106244

Gille, F. and Brall, C. (2021b) 'Limits of data anonymity: lack of public awareness risks trust in health system activities', *Life Sciences, Society and Policy*, 17: 7. https://doi.org/10.1186/s40504-021-00115-9

Gille, F. and Vayena, E. (2021) 'How private individuals maintain privacy and govern their own health data cooperative: MIDATA in Switzerland', in B.M. Frischmann, K.J. Strandburg and M.R. Sanfilippo (eds) *Governing Privacy in Knowledge Commons*, Cambridge: Cambridge University Press (Cambridge Studies on Governing Knowledge Commons), pp 53–69. https://doi.org/10.1017/9781108749978.003

Gille, F., Smith, S. and Mays, N. (2014) 'Why public trust in health care systems matters and deserves greater research attention', *Journal of Health Services Research & Policy*, 20(1), pp 62–4. https://doi.org/10.1177/1355819614543161

Gille, F., Smith, S. and Mays, N. (2017) 'Towards a broader conceptualisation of "public trust" in the health care system', *Social Theory & Health*, 15(1), pp 25–43. https://doi.org/10.1057/s41285-016-0017-y

Gille, F., Axler, R. and Blasimme, A. (2020) 'Transparency about governance contributes to biobanks' trustworthiness: call for action', *Biopreservation and Biobanking*, 19(1), pp 83–5. https://doi.org/10.1089/bio.2020.0057

Gille, F., Jobin, A. and Ienca, M. (2020) 'What we talk about when we talk about trust: theory of trust for AI in healthcare', *Intelligence-Based Medicine*, 1–2, p 100001. https://doi.org/10.1016/j.ibmed.2020.100001

Gille, F., Smith, S. and Mays, N. (2020) 'What is public trust in the healthcare system? A new conceptual framework developed from qualitative data in England', *Social Theory & Health*, 19(1), pp 1–20. https://doi.org/10.1057/s41285-020-00129-x

Gille, F., Vayena, E. and Blasimme, A. (2020) 'Future-proofing biobanks' governance', *European Journal of Human Genetics*, 28, pp 989–96. https://doi.org/10.1038/s41431-020-0646-4

Gille, F., Smith, S. and Mays, N. (2022) 'Evidence-based guiding principles to build public trust in personal data use in health systems', *DIGITAL HEALTH*, 8, p 20552076221111947. https://doi.org/10.1177/20552076221111947

Gilson, L. (2003) 'Trust and the development of health care as a social institution', *Social Science & Medicine*, 56(7), pp 1453–68. https://doi.org/10.1016/s0277-9536(02)00142-9

Gilson, L. (2006) 'Trust in health care: theoretical perspectives and research needs', *Journal of Health Organization and Management,* 20(5), pp 359–75. https://doi.org/10.1108/14777260610701768

Gilson, L., Palmer, N. and Schneider, H. (2005) 'Trust and health worker performance: exploring a conceptual framework using South African evidence', *Social Science & Medicine: Building Trust and Value in Health Systems in Low- and Middle-Income Countries*, 61(7), pp 1418–29. https://doi.org/10.1016/j.socscimed.2004.11.062

Giritli Nygren, K. and Olofsson, A. (2021) 'Swedish exceptionalism, herd immunity and the welfare state: a media analysis of struggles over the nature and legitimacy of the COVID-19 pandemic strategy in Sweden', *Current Sociology*, 69(4), pp 529–46. https://doi.org/10.1177/0011392121990025

Goertzel, T. (1994) 'Belief in conspiracy theories', *Political Psychology*, 15(4), pp 731–42. https://doi.org/10.2307/3791630

Goodnight, G.T. and Poulakos, J. (1981) 'Conspiracy rhetoric: from pragmatism to fantasy in public discourse', *Western Journal of Speech Communication*, 45(4), pp 299–316. https://doi.org/10.1080/10570318109374052

Gopichandran, V. (2017) 'Public trust in vaccination: an analytical framework', *Indian Journal of Medical Ethics*, 2(2), 98–104. https://doi.org/10.20529/IJME.2017.024

Gopichandran, V., Subramaniam, S. and Kalsingh, M.J. (2020) 'COVID-19 pandemic: a litmus test of trust in the health system', *Asian Bioethics Review*, 12(2), pp 213–21. https://doi.org/10.1007/s41649-020-00122-6

Goudge, J. and Gilson, L. (2005) 'How can trust be investigated? Drawing lessons from past experience', *Social Science & Medicine*, 61(7), pp 1439–51. https://doi.org/10.1016/j.socscimed.2004.11.071

Green, J. and Browne, J. (2005) *Principles of Social Research*, Open University Press.

Greenhalgh, T. et al (2021) 'Ten scientific reasons in support of airborne transmission of SARS-CoV-2', *The Lancet*, 397(10285), pp 1603–5. https://doi.org/10.1016/S0140-6736(21)00869-2

Groenewegen, P.P., Hansen, J. and Jong, J.D. de (2019) 'Trust in times of health reform', *Health Policy*, 123(3), pp 281–7. https://doi.org/10.1016/j.healthpol.2018.11.016

Guntuku, S.C. et al (2021) 'Twitter discourse reveals geographical and temporal variation in concerns about COVID-19 vaccines in the United States', *Vaccine*, 39(30), pp 4034–8. https://doi.org/10.1016/j.vaccine.2021.06.014

Haasteren, A. van et al (2019) 'Development of the mHealth App trustworthiness checklist', *DIGITAL HEALTH*, 5, p 2055207619886463. https://doi.org/10.1177/2055207619886463

Habermas, J. (1995) *Theorie des kommunikativen Handelns* (1. Aufl.), *Suhrkamp Taschenbuch Wissenschaft*, Berlin: Suhrkamp.

Hafen, E., Kossmann, D. and Brand, A. (2014) 'Health data cooperatives – citizen empowerment', *Methods of Information in Medicine*, 53(02), pp 82–6. https://doi.org/10.3414/ME13-02-0051

Hall, M.A. et al (2002) 'Measuring patients' trust in their primary care providers', *Medical Care Research and Review*, 59(3), pp 293–318. https://doi.org/10.1177/1077558702059003004

Halpern, D. et al (2019) 'From belief in conspiracy theories to trust in others: which factors influence exposure, believing and sharing fake news', in G. Meiselwitz (ed) *Social Computing and Social Media. Design, Human Behavior and Analytics*, Cham: Springer International Publishing, pp 217–32.

Hanson, C. et al (2021) 'National health governance, science and the media: drivers of COVID-19 responses in Germany, Sweden and the UK in 2020', *BMJ Global Health*, 6(12), p e006691. https://doi.org/10.1136/bmjgh-2021-006691

Harachi, T.W. et al (2006) 'Examining equivalence of concepts and measures in diverse samples', *Prevention Science*, 7(4), pp 359–68. https://doi.org/10.1007/s11121-006-0039-0

Hardin, R. (1993) 'The street-level epistemology of trust', *Politics & Society*, 21(4), pp 505–29.

Hardin, R. (1999) 'Do we want trust in government?', in M.E. Warren (ed) *Democracy and Trust*, Cambridge: Cambridge University Press, pp 22–41. https://doi.org/10.1017/CBO9780511659959.002

Hardin, R. (2006) *Trust, Key Concepts*, Cambridge: Polity.

Hardin, R. (2009) 'Compliance, consent, and legitimacy', in C. Boix and S.C. Stokes (eds) *The Oxford Handbook of Comparative Politics*, Oxford University Press, pp 236–55. https://doi.org/10.1093/oxfordhb/9780199566020.003.0010

Harpe, S.E. (2015) 'How to analyze Likert and other rating scale data', *Currents in Pharmacy Teaching and Learning*, 7(6), pp 836–50. https://doi.org/10.1016/j.cptl.2015.08.001

Harrison, J., Innes, R. and Zwanenberg, T. van (eds) (2003) *Rebuilding Trust in Healthcare*, Abingdon: Radcliffe Medical Press.

Hartmann, M. (1994) *Die Praxis des Vertrauens* (1st edn), Berlin: Suhrkamp.

Hartmann, M. (2015) 'On the concept of basic trust', *BEHEMOTH – A Journal on Civilisation*, 8(1), pp 5–23. https://doi.org/10.6094/BEHEMOTH.2015.8.1.850

Haselhuhn, M.P., Schweitzer, M.E. and Wood, A.M. (2010) 'How implicit beliefs influence trust recovery', *Psychological Science*, 21(5), pp 645–8. https://doi.org/10.1177/0956797610367752

Hawkins, A.K. and O'Doherty, K. (2010) 'Biobank governance: a lesson in trust', *New Genetics and Society*, 29(3), pp 311–27. https://doi.org/10.1080/14636778.2010.507487

Hays, R. and Daker-White, G. (2015) 'The care.data consensus? A qualitative analysis of opinions expressed on Twitter', *BMC Public Health*, 15, p 838. https://doi.org/10.1186/s12889-015-2180-9

Heijlen, R. and Crompvoets, J. (2021) 'Open health data: Mapping the ecosystem', *DIGITAL HEALTH*, 7, p 20552076211050170. https://doi.org/10.1177/20552076211050167

Heinecke, S. (2019) 'The game of trust: reflections on truth and trust in a shifting media ecosystem', in T. Osburg and S. Heinecke (eds) *Media Trust in a Digital World: Communication at Crossroads*, Cham: Springer International Publishing, pp 3–13. https://doi.org/10.1007/978-3-030-30774-5_1

Hensel, L. et al (2022) 'Global behaviors, perceptions, and the emergence of social norms at the onset of the COVID-19 pandemic', *Journal of Economic Behavior & Organization*, 193, pp 473–96. https://doi.org/10.1016/j.jebo.2021.11.015

Hieronymi, P. (2008) 'The reasons of trust', *Australasian Journal of Philosophy*, 86(2), pp 213–36. https://doi.org/10.1080/00048400801886496

Horvath, L., Banducci, S. and James, O. (2022) 'Citizens' attitudes to contact tracing apps', *Journal of Experimental Political Science*, 9(1), pp 118–30. https://doi.org/10.1017/XPS.2020.30

Høyer, H.C. and Mønness, E. (2016) 'Trust in public institutions – spillover and bandwidth', *Journal of Trust Research*, 6(2), pp 151–66. https://doi.org/10.1080/21515581.2016.1156546

Ienca, M. et al (2018) 'Considerations for ethics review of big data health research: a scoping review', *PLOS ONE*, 13(10), p e0204937. https://doi.org/10.1371/journal.pone.0204937

Ienca, M. and Vayena, E. (2020) 'On the responsible use of digital data to tackle the COVID-19 pandemic', *Nature Medicine*, 26(4), pp 463–4. https://doi.org/10.1038/s41591-020-0832-5

Ipsos (2022) 'Ipsos'. Available from: https://www.ipsos.com/en-us (Accessed: 12 October 2022).

Ipsos Mori (2019) *Trust: the truth?* Ipsos Mori, [online]. 18 September. Available from: https://www.ipsos.com/ipsos-mori/en-uk/ipsos-thinks-trust-truth (Accessed: 2 March 2023).

Jackson, J. and Gau, J.M. (2016) 'Carving up concepts? Differentiating between trust and legitimacy in public attitudes towards legal authority', in E. Shockley et al (eds) *Interdisciplinary Perspectives on Trust: Towards Theoretical and Methodological Integration*. Cham: Springer International Publishing, pp 49–69. https://doi.org/10.1007/978-3-319-22261-5_3

Jacobs, A.K. (2005) 'Rebuilding an enduring trust in medicine: a global mandate: Presidential address American Heart Association Scientific Sessions 2004', *Circulation*, 111(25), pp 3494–8. https://doi.org/10.1161/CIRCULATIONAHA. 105.166277

Jansen, N.E. et al (2022) 'Changing to an opt out system for organ donation – reflections from England and Netherlands', *Transplant International*, 35. https://doi.org/10.3389/ti.2022.10466

Jenkins, R. (2008) 'The ambiguity of Europe: "Identity crisis" or "situation normal"?', *European Societies*, 10(2), pp 153–76. https://doi.org/10.1080/14616690701835253

Jobin, A., Ienca, M. and Vayena, E. (2019) 'The global landscape of AI ethics guidelines', *Nature Machine Intelligence*, 1(9), pp 389–99. https://doi.org/10.1038/s42256-019-0088-2

Johnson, N.D. and Mislin, A.A. (2011) 'Trust games: a meta-analysis', *Journal of Economic Psychology*, 32(5), pp 865–89. https://doi.org/10.1016/j.joep.2011.05.007

Jolley, D. and Douglas, K.M. (2014) 'The effects of anti-vaccine conspiracy theories on vaccination intentions', *PLOS ONE*, 9(2), p e89177. https://doi.org/10.1371/journal.pone.0089177

Jovančević, A. and Milićević, N. (2020) 'Optimism-pessimism, conspiracy theories and general trust as factors contributing to COVID-19 related behavior – a cross-cultural study', Personality and Individual Differences, 167, p 110216. https://doi.org/10.1016/j.paid.2020.110216

Kaasa, A. and Andriani, L. (2022) 'Determinants of institutional trust: the role of cultural context', *Journal of Institutional Economics*, 18(1), pp 45–65. https://doi.org/10.1017/S1744137421000199

Kalkman, S. et al (2022) 'Patients' and public views and attitudes towards the sharing of health data for research: a narrative review of the empirical evidence', *Journal of Medical Ethics*, 48(1), p 3. https://doi.org/10.1136/medethics-2019-105651

Kc, S. et al (2022) 'Factors associated with the opposition to COVID-19 vaccination certificates: a multi-country observational study from Asia', *Travel Medicine and Infectious Disease*, 48, p 102358. https://doi.org/10.1016/j.tmaid.2022.102358

Keating, N.L. et al (2004) 'Patient characteristics and experiences associated with trust in specialist physicians', *Archives of Internal Medicine*, 164(9), pp 1015–20. https://doi.org/10.1001/archinte.164.9.1015

Khodarahmi, E. (2009) 'Crisis management', *Disaster Prevention and Management: An International Journal*, 18(5), pp 523–8. https://doi.org/10.1108/09653560911003714

Kickbusch, I. (2019) 'Health promotion 4.0', *Health Promotion International*, 34(2), pp 179–81. https://doi.org/10.1093/heapro/daz022

Kohn, L.T., Corrigan, J. and Donaldson, M.S. (eds) (2000) *To Err is Human: Building a Safer Health System*, Washington, DC: National Academy Press.

Koltko-Rivera, M.E. (2004) 'The psychology of worldviews', *Review of General Psychology*, 8(1), pp 3–58. https://doi.org/10.1037/1089-2680.8.1.3

Krause, N.M. et al (2020) 'Fact-checking as risk communication: the multi-layered risk of misinformation in times of COVID-19', *Journal of Risk Research*, 23(7–8), pp 1052–9. https://doi.org/10.1080/13669877.2020.1756385

Kroeger, F. (2017) 'Facework: creating trust in systems, institutions and organisations', *Cambridge Journal of Economics*, 41(2), pp 487–514. https://doi.org/10.1093/cje/bew038

Krouwel, A. et al (2017) 'Does extreme political ideology predict conspiracy beliefs, economic evaluations and political trust? Evidence from Sweden', *Journal of Social and Political Psychology*, 5(2), pp 435–62. https://doi.org/10.5964/jspp.v5i2.745

Kuhn, S.A.K. et al (2021) 'Coronavirus conspiracy beliefs in the German-speaking general population: endorsement rates and links to reasoning biases and paranoia', *Psychological Medicine*, 52(16), pp 4162–76. https://doi.org/10.1017/S0033291721001124

Kunitoki, K. et al (2021) 'Access to HPV vaccination in Japan: Increasing social trust to regain vaccine confidence', *Vaccine*, 39(41), pp 6104–10. https://doi.org/10.1016/j.vaccine.2021.08.085

Kurten, S. and Beullens, K. (2021) '#Coronavirus: monitoring the Belgian Twitter discourse on the Severe Acute Respiratory Syndrome Coronavirus 2 pandemic', *Cyberpsychology, Behavior, and Social Networking*, 24(2), pp 117–22. https://doi.org/10.1089/cyber.2020.0341

Larson, H.J. et al (2011) 'Addressing the vaccine confidence gap', *The Lancet*, 378(9790), pp 526–35. http://dx.doi.org/10.1016/S0140-6736(11)60678-8

Larson, H.J. et al (2016) 'The state of vaccine confidence 2016: Global insights through a 67-country survey', *EBioMedicine*, 12, pp 295–301. https://doi.org/10.1016/j.ebiom.2016.08.042

Larson, H.J. (2016) 'Vaccine trust and the limits of information', *Science*, 353(6305), p 1207. https://www.science.org/doi/10.1126/science.aah6190

Larson, H.J. et al (2018) 'Measuring trust in vaccination: A systematic review', *Human Vaccines & Immunotherapeutics*, 14(7), pp 1599–1609. https://doi.org/10.1080/21645515.2018.1459252

Laugharne, R. et al (2012) 'Trust, choice and power in mental health care: Experiences of patients with psychosis', *International Journal of Social Psychiatry*, 58(5), pp 496–504. https://doi.org/10.1177/0020764011408658

Lawler, M. et al (2018) 'A roadmap for restoring trust in Big Data', *The Lancet Oncology*, 19(8), pp 1014–15. https://doi.org/10.1016/S1470-2045(18)30425-X

Lee, K. (2009) 'How the Hong Kong government lost the public trust in SARS: insights for government communication in a health crisis', *Public Relations Review*, 35(1), pp 74–6. https://doi.org/10.1016/j.pubrev.2008.06.003

Levine, J.S. (2004) 'Trust: can we create the time?', *Archives of Internal Medicine*, 164(9), pp 930–2. https://doi.org/10.1001/archinte.164.9.930

Levine, L. (2019) 'Digital trust and cooperation with an integrative digital social contract', *Journal of Business Ethics*, 160(2), pp 393–407. https://doi.org/10.1007/s10551-019-04201-z

Li, H. et al (2014) 'Examining the decision to use standalone personal health record systems as a trust-enabled fair social contract', *Decision Support Systems*, 57, pp 376–86. https://doi.org/10.1016/j.dss.2012.10.043

Limaye, R.J. et al (2020) 'Building trust while influencing online COVID-19 content in the social media world', *The Lancet Digital Health*, 2(6), pp e277–e278. https://doi.org/10.1016/S2589-7500(20)30084-4

Lipset, S.M. (1959) 'Some social requisites of democracy: economic development and political legitimacy', *American Political Science Review*, 53(1), pp 69–105. https://doi.org/10.2307/1951731

Liu, H. and Priest, S. (2009) 'Understanding public support for stem cell research: media communication, interpersonal communication and trust in key actors', *Public Understanding of Science*, 18(6), pp 704–18. https://doi.org/10.1177/0963662508097625

Liu, J.H. et al (2018) 'The Global Trust Inventory as a "proxy measure" for social capital: measurement and impact in 11 democratic societies', *Journal of Cross-Cultural Psychology*, 49(5), pp 789–810. https://doi.org/10.1177/0022022118766619

Liu, P.L. and Jiang, S. (2021) 'Patient-centered communication mediates the relationship between health information acquisition and patient trust in physicians: a five-year comparison in China', *Health Communication*, 36(2), pp 207–16. https://doi.org/10.1080/10410236.2019.1673948

Liu, Y. et al (2022) 'What matters: non-pharmaceutical interventions for COVID-19 in Europe', *Antimicrobial Resistance & Infection Control*, 11: 3. https://doi.org/10.1186/s13756-021-01039-x

Locock, L. and Boylan, A.-M.R. (2016) 'Biosamples as gifts? How participants in biobanking projects talk about donation', *Health Expectations: An International Journal of Public Participation in Health Care and Health Policy*, 19(4), pp 805–16. https://doi.org/10.1111/hex.12376

Lohr, K.N. (2002) 'Assessing health status and quality-of-life instruments: attributes and review criteria', *Quality of Life Research*, 11(3), pp 193–205. https://doi.org/10.1023/A:1015291021312

Lounsbury, O. et al (2021) 'Opening a "can of worms" to explore the public's hopes and fears about health care data sharing: qualitative study', *Journal of Medical Internet Research*, 23(2), p e22744. https://doi.org/10.2196/22744

Luhmann, N. (1988) 'Familiarity, confidence, trust: problems and perspectives', in D. Gambetta (ed) *Trust: Making and Breaking Cooperative Relations*, New York: Blackwell.

Luhmann, N. (2009) *Vertrauen: ein Mechanismus der Reduktion sozialer Komplexität* (4. Aufl.), *UTB für Wissenschaft Soziologie fachübergreifend,* Stuttgart: Lucius & Lucius.

Luhmann, N. (2017) *Trust and Power*, M. King and C. Morgner (eds), H. Davies, J. Raffan and K. Rooney (trans), Cambridge: Polity Press.

Lunshof, J.E. et al (2008) 'From genetic privacy to open consent', *Nature Reviews Genetics*, 9, pp 406–11. https://doi.org/10.1038/nrg2360

Luo, W. and Najdawi, M. (2004) 'Trust-building measures: a review of consumer health portals', *Communications of the ACM*, 47(1), pp 108–13. https://doi.org/10.1145/962081.962089

MacKenzie, S.B. (2003) 'The dangers of poor construct conceptualization', *Journal of the Academy of Marketing Science*, 31(3), pp 323–6. https://doi.org/10.1177/009207030303 1003011

Makowska, M., Boguszewski, R. and Podkowińska, M. (2022) 'Trust in medicine as a factor conditioning behaviors recommended by healthcare experts during the COVID-19 pandemic in Poland', *International Journal of Environmental Research and Public Health*, 19(1), p 605. https://doi.org/10.3390/ijerph19010605

Marcon, A.R. et al (2022) 'Web-based perspectives of deemed consent organ donation legislation in Nova Scotia: thematic analysis of commentary in Facebook groups', *JMIR Infodemiology*, 2(2), p e38242. https://doi.org/10.2196/38242

Mari, S. et al (2021) 'Conspiracy theories and institutional trust: examining the role of uncertainty avoidance and active social media use', Political Psychology, 43(2), pp 277–96. https://doi.org/10.1111/pops.12754

Marques, M.D., Douglas, K.M. and Jolley, D. (2022) 'Practical recommendations to communicate with patients about health-related conspiracy theories', *Medical Journal of Australia*, 216(8), pp 381–4. https://doi.org/10.5694/mja2.51475

Martin, S. et al (2020) '"Vaccines for pregnant women …?! Absurd" – Mapping maternal vaccination discourse and stance on social media over six months', *Vaccine*, 38(42), pp 6627–37. https://doi.org/10.1016/j.vaccine.2020.07.072

Mattila, M. and Rapeli, L. (2018) 'Just sick of it? Health and political trust in Western Europe', *European Journal of Political Research*, 57(1), pp 116–34. https://doi.org/10.1111/1475-6765.12218

Mattocks, K.M. et al (2017) 'Mistrust and endorsement of human immunodeficiency virus conspiracy theories among human immunodeficiency virus–infected African American veterans', *Military Medicine*, 182(11–12), pp e2073–e2079. https://doi.org/10.7205/MILMED-D-17-00078

May, T. (2005) 'Public communication, risk perception, and the viability of preventive vaccination against communicable diseases', *Bioethics*, 19(4), pp 407–21. https://doi.org/10.1111/j.1467-8519.2005.00452.x

McGraw, D. et al (2009) 'Privacy as an enabler, not an impediment: building trust into health information exchange', *Health Affairs*, 28(2), pp 416–27. https://doi.org/10.1377/hlthaff.28.2.416

McKenzie-McHarg, A. (2020) 'Conceptual history and conspiracy theory', in M. Butter and P. Knight (eds) *Routledge Handbook of Conspiracy Theories*, Abingdon: Routledge, pp 16–27.

Mechanic, D. (1996) 'Changing medical organization and the erosion of trust', *The Milbank Quarterly*, 74(2), pp 171–89. https://doi.org/10.2307/3350245

Mechanic, D. (1998) 'The functions and limitations of trust in the provision of medical care', *Journal of Health Politics, Policy and Law*, 23(4), pp 661–86. https://doi.org/10.1215/03616878-23-4-661

Mensah, I.K. and Adams, S. (2020) 'A comparative analysis of the impact of political trust on the adoption of e-government services', *International Journal of Public Administration*, 43(8), pp 682–96. https://doi.org/10.1080/01900692.2019.1645687

Meszaros, J. and Ho, C. (2019) 'Building trust and transparency? Challenges of the opt-out system and the secondary use of health data in England', *Medical Law International*, 19(2–3), pp 159–81. https://doi.org/10.1177/0968533219879975

Meszaros, J., Ho, C. and Corrales Compagnucci, M. (2020) 'Nudging consent and the new opt-out system to the processing of health data in England', in M. Corrales Compagnucci et al (eds) *Legal Tech and the New Sharing Economy*, Singapore: Springer Singapore, pp 93–113. https://doi.org/10.1007/978-981-15-1350-3_5

Meyer, S. et al (2008) 'Trust in the health system: an analysis and extension of the social theories of Giddens and Luhmann', *Health Sociology Review*, 17(2), pp 177–86. https://doi.org/10.5172/hesr.451.17.2.177

Meyer, S.B. and Ward, P.R. (2013) 'Differentiating between trust and dependence of patients with coronary heart disease: furthering the sociology of trust', *Health, Risk & Society*, 15(3), pp 279–93. https://doi.org/10.1080/13698575.2013.776017.

Middleton, B. et al (2013) 'Enhancing patient safety and quality of care by improving the usability of electronic health record systems: recommendations from AMIA', *Journal of the American Medical Informatics Association*, 20(e1), pp e2–e8. https://doi.org/10.1136/amiajnl-2012-001458

Milne, R. et al (2019) 'Trust in genomic data sharing among members of the general public in the UK, USA, Canada and Australia', *Human Genetics*, 138(11), pp 1237–46. https://doi.org/10.1007/s00439-019-02062-0

Misztal, B.A. (1996) *Trust in Modern Societies*, Hoboken: Blackwell Publishers Inc.

Moberly, T. (2014) 'Care.data must become an opt-in system, say doctors', *BMJ (Clinical Research Edition)*, 348, p g4284.

Mohseni, M. and Lindstrom, M. (2007) 'Social capital, trust in the health-care system and self-rated health: the role of access to health care in a population-based study', *Social Science & Medicine*, 64(7), pp 1373–83. https://doi.org/10.1016/j.socscimed.2006.11.023

Möllering, G. (2001) 'The nature of trust: from Georg Simmel to a theory of expectation, interpretation and suspension', *Sociology*, 35(2), pp 403–20. https://doi.org/10.1177/S003803850100019

Montinola, G.R. (2004) 'Corruption, distrust, and the deterioration of the rule of law', in R. Hardin (ed) *Distrust*, Russell Sage Foundation, pp 298–324. Available from: http://www.jstor.org/stable/10.7758/9781610442695.16 (Accessed: 5 November 2022).

Moodley, K. (2017) 'Legitimacy, trust and stakeholder engagement: biobanking in South Africa', *Asian Bioethics Review*, 9(4), pp 325–34. https://doi.org/10.1007/s41649-017-0035-7

Morley, J. et al (2020) 'Ethical guidelines for COVID-19 tracing apps', *Nature*, 582(7810), pp 29–31. https://doi.org/10.1038/d41586-020-01578-0

Muirhead, R. and Rosenblum, N.L. (2016) 'Speaking truth to conspiracy: partisanship and trust', *Critical Review*, 28(1), pp 63–88. https://doi.org/10.1080/08913811.2016.1173981

Muller, S.H.A. et al (2021) 'The social licence for data-intensive health research: towards co-creation, public value and trust', *BMC Medical Ethics*, 22(1), p 110. https://doi.org/10.1186/s12910-021-00677-5

Muric, G., Wu, Y. and Ferrara, E. (2021) 'COVID-19 vaccine hesitancy on social media: building a public Twitter data set of antivaccine content, accine misinformation, and conspiracies', *JMIR Public Health and Surveillance*, 7(11), p e30642. https://doi.org/10.2196/30642

Murray, C.J. and Frenk, J. (2000) 'A framework for assessing the performance of health systems', *Bulletin of the World Health Organization*, 78(6), pp 717–31.

Musgrove, A.T. et al (2018) 'Real or fake? Resources for teaching college students how to identify fake news', *College & Undergraduate Libraries*, 25(3), pp 243–60. https://doi.org/10.1080/10691316.2018.1480444

Narayana Samy, G., Ahmad, R. and Ismail, Z. (2010) 'Security threats categories in healthcare information systems', *Health Informatics Journal*, 16(3), pp 201–9. https://doi.org/10.1177/1460458210377468

Natalier, K. and Willis, K. (2008) 'Taking responsibility or averting risk? A socio-cultural approach to risk and trust in private health insurance decisions', *Health, Risk & Society*, 10(4), pp 399–411. https://doi.org/10.1080/13698570802167413

National Data Guardian (2016) *Review of Data Security, Consent and Opt-Outs*, p 59. Available from: https://www.gov.uk/government/uploads/system/uploads/attachment_data/file/535024/data-security-review.PDF (Accessed: 12 July 2023).

National Data Guardian (2020) The Eight Caldicott Principles. Available from: https://assets.publishing.service.gov.uk/government/uploads/system/uploads/attachment_data/file/942217/Eight_Caldicott_Principles_08.12.20.pdf (Accessed: 20 October 2022).

Netemeyer, R.G. et al (2020) 'Health literacy, health numeracy, and trust in doctor: Effects on key patient health outcomes', *Journal of Consumer Affairs*, 54(1), pp 3–42. https://doi.org/10.1111/joca.12267

Neuberger, C., Langenohl, S. and Nuernbergk, C. (2015) *Social Media und Journalismus* (2te unveränderte Auflage), Düsseldorf: LfM-Dokumentation, Band 50.

Newton, J.D. (2011) 'How does the general public view posthumous organ donation? A meta-synthesis of the qualitative literature', *BMC Public Health*, 11(1), p 791. https://doi.org/10.1186/1471-2458-11-791

Ngai, C.S.B. et al (2022) 'Exploring the relationship between trust-building strategies and public engagement on social media during the COVID-19 outbreak', *Health Communication*, pp 1–17. https://doi.org/10.1080/10410236.2022.2055261

Nieminen, T. et al (2013) 'Social capital, health behaviours and health: a population-based associational study', *BMC Public Health*, 13: 613. https://doi.org/10.1186/1471-2458-13-613

Nikodem, K., Ćurković, M. and Borovečki, A. (2022) 'Trust in the healthcare system and physicians in Croatia: A survey of the general population', *International Journal of Environmental Research and Public Health*, 19(2). https://doi.org/10.3390/ijerph19020993

Noyon, L., de Keijser, J.W. and Crijns, J.H. (2020) 'Legitimacy and public opinion: a five-step model', *International Journal of Law in Context*, 16(4), pp 390–402. https://doi.org/10.1017/S1744552320000403

Nundy, S., Montgomery, T. and Wachter, R.M. (2019) 'Promoting trust between patients and physicians in the era of Artificial Intelligence', *JAMA*, 322(6), pp 497–8. https://doi.org/10.1001/jama.2018.20563

Nutbeam, D. (2000) 'Health literacy as a public health goal: a challenge for contemporary health education and communication strategies into the 21st century', *Health Promotion International*, 15(3), pp 259–67. https://doi.org/10.1093/heapro/15.3.259

Nwebonyi, N., Silva, S. and de Freitas, C. (2022) 'Public views about involvement in decision-making on health data sharing, access, use and reuse: The importance of trust in science and other institutions', *Frontiers in Public Health*, 10, p 852971. https://doi.org/10.3389/fpubh.2022.852971

Nys, T. (2015) 'Autonomy, trust, and respect', *Journal of Medicine and Philosophy*, 41(1), pp 10–24. https://doi.org/10.1093/jmp/jhv036

OECD (Organisation for Economic Co-operation and Development) (2017) *OECD Guidelines on Measuring Trust*, Paris: OECD Publishing. https://doi.org/10.1787/9789264278219-en

OECD (2018) *Bridging the Digital Gender Divide*. Available from: https://www.oecd.org/digital/bridging-the-digital-gender-divide.pdf (Accessed: 2 March 2023).

OECD (2022) 'Trust in government', OECD, [online]. https://doi.org/10.1787/1de9675e-en

Office of the U.S. Surgeon General (2021) *A Community Toolkit for Addressing Health Misinformation*. Available from: https://www.hhs.gov/sites/default/files/health-misinformation-toolkit-english.pdf (Accessed: 12 July 2023).

Oliver, J.E. and Wood, T. (2014) 'Medical conspiracy theories and health behaviors in the United States', *JAMA Internal Medicine*, 174(5), pp 817–18. https://doi.org/10.1001/jamainternmed.2014.190

Oliver, J.E. and Wood, T.J. (2014) 'Conspiracy theories and the paranoid style(s) of mass opinion', *American Journal of Political Science*, 58(4), pp 952–66. https://doi.org/10.1111/ajps.12084

O'Neill, O. (2002) *Autonomy and Trust in Bioethics (Gifford Lectures)*, Cambridge: Cambridge University Press.

O'Neill, O. (2003) *A Question of Trust* (repr), Cambridge: Cambridge University Press.

O'Neill, O. (2020) 'Trust and accountability in a digital age', *Philosophy*, 14 October 2019 edn, 95(1), pp 3–17. https://doi.org/DOI: 10.1017/S0031819119000457

Østergaard, L.R. (2015) 'Trust matters: A narrative literature review of the role of trust in health care systems in sub-Saharan Africa', *Global Public Health*, 10(9), pp 1046–59. https://doi.org/10.1080/17441692.2015.1019538

Ostherr, K. et al (2017) 'Trust and privacy in the context of user-generated health data', *Big Data & Society*, 4(1), p 2053951717704673. https://doi.org/10.1177/2053951717704673

O'Sullivan, S., Healy, A.E. and Breen, M.J. (2014) 'Political legitimacy in Ireland during economic crisis: insights from the European social survey', *Irish Political Studies*, 29(4), pp 547–72. https://doi.org/10.1080/07907184.2014.942645

Ozawa, S. and Sripad, P. (2013) 'How do you measure trust in the health system? A systematic review of the literature', *Social Science & Medicine*, 91, pp 10–14. https://doi.org/10.1016/j.socsci med.2013.05.005

Ozawa, S., Paina, L. and Qiu, M. (2016) 'Exploring pathways for building trust in vaccination and strengthening health system resilience', *BMC Health Services Research*, 16(7), p 639. https://doi.org/10.1186/s12913-016-1867-7

Pagliaro, S. et al (2021) 'Trust predicts COVID-19 prescribed and discretionary behavioral intentions in 23 countries', *PLOS ONE*, 16(3), p e0248334. https://doi.org/10.1371/journal.pone.0248334

Papakostas, A. (2012) *Civilizing the Public Sphere: Distrust, Trust and Corruption*, Palgrave Studies in European Political Sociology, London: Palgrave Macmillan UK. https://doi.org/10.1007/978-1-137-03042-9

Parsons, R. and Moffat, K. (2014) 'Constructing the meaning of social licence', *Social Epistemology*, 28(3–4), pp 340–63. https://doi.org/10.1080/02691728.2014.922645

Pearson, S.D. and Raeke, L.H. (2000) 'Patients' trust in physicians: many theories, few measures, and little data', *Journal of General Internal Medicine*, 15(7), pp 509–13. https://doi.org/10.1046/j.1525-1497.2000.11002.x

Pérez-Escoda, A. et al (2020) 'Social networks' engagement during the COVID-19 pandemic in Spain: health media vs. healthcare professionals', *International Journal of Environmental Research and Public Health*, 17(14), p 5261. https://doi.org/10.3390/ijerph1 7145261

Pergert, P. and Lützén, K. (2012) 'Balancing truth-telling in the preservation of hope: a relational ethics approach', *Nursing Ethics*, 19(1), pp 21–9. https://doi.org/10.1177/0969733011418551

Perron, B.E. and Gillespie, D.F. (2015) *Key Concepts in Measurement*, New York: Oxford University Press. https://doi.org/10.1093/acprof:oso/9780199855483.001.0001

Peters, D. and Youssef, F.F. (2016) 'Public trust in the healthcare system in a developing country', *The International Journal of Health Planning and Management*, 31(2), pp 227–41. https://doi.org/10.1002/hpm.2280

Petersen, A. (2005) 'Securing our genetic health: engendering trust in UK Biobank', *Sociology of Health & Illness*, 27(2), pp 271–92. https://doi.org/10.1111/j.1467-9566.2005.00442.x

Pilgrim, D., Tomasini, F. and Vassilev, I. (2010) *Examining Trust in Healthcare A Multidisciplinary Perspective*, London: Palgrave Macmillan.

Platt, J. and Kardia, S. (2015) 'Public trust in health information sharing: implications for biobanking and electronic health record systems', *Journal of Personalized Medicine*, 5(1), pp 3–21. https://doi.org/10.3390/jpm5010003

Platt, J.E., Jacobson, P.D. and Kardia, S.L.R. (2018) 'Public trust in health information sharing: a measure of system trust', *Health Services Research*, 53(2), pp 824–45. https://doi.org/10.1111/1475-6773.12654

Platt, J., Raj, M. and Kardia, S.L.R. (2019) 'The public's trust and information brokers in health care, public health and research', *Journal of Health Organization and Management*, 33(7/8), pp 929–48. https://doi.org/10.1108/JHOM-11-2018-0332

Plohl, N. and Musil, B. (2020) 'Modeling compliance with COVID-19 prevention guidelines: the critical role of trust in science', *Psychology, Health and Medicine*, 26(1), pp 1–12. https://doi.org/10.1080/13548506.2020.1772988

Pummerer, L. et al (2021) 'Conspiracy theories and their societal effects during the COVID-19 pandemic', *Social Psychological and Personality Science*, 13(1), pp 49–59. https://doi.org/10.1177/19485506211000217

Puri, N. et al (2020) 'Social media and vaccine hesitancy: new updates for the era of COVID-19 and globalized infectious diseases', *Human Vaccines & Immunotherapeutics*, 16(11), pp 2586–93. https://doi.org/10.1080/21645515.2020.1780846

Qiao, Y., Asan, O. and Montague, E. (2015) 'Factors associated with patient trust in electronic health records used in primary care settings', *Health Policy and Technology*, 4(4), pp 357–63. https://doi.org/10.1016/j.hlpt.2015.08.001

Quinn, S.C. et al (2013) 'Exploring communication, trust in government, and vaccination intention later in the 2009 H1N1 pandemic: results of a national survey', *Biosecurity and Bioterrorism: Biodefense Strategy, Practice, and Science*, 11(2), pp 96–106. https://doi.org/10.1089/bsp.2012.0048

Randolph, S.D. et al (2022) 'Adaptive leadership in clinical encounters with women living with HIV', *BMC Women's Health*, 22: 217. https://doi.org/10.1186/s12905-022-01810-1

Reeve, B.B. et al (2013) 'ISOQOL recommends minimum standards for patient-reported outcome measures used in patient-centered outcomes and comparative effectiveness research', *Quality of Life Research*, 22(8), pp 1889–1905. https://doi.org/10.1007/s11136-012-0344-y

Rekker, R. and Harteveld, E. (2022) 'Understanding factual belief polarization: the role of trust, political sophistication, and affective polarization', Acta Politica [Preprint]. https://doi.org/10.1057/s41269-022-00265-4

Robison, L.J., Schmid, A.A. and Siles, M.E. (2002) 'Is social capital really capital?', *Review of Social Economy*, 60(1), pp 1–21. https://doi.org/10.1080/00346760110127074

Rosenbaum, S. (2010) 'Data governance and stewardship: designing data stewardship entities and advancing data access', *Health Services Research*, 45(5p2), pp 1442–55. https://doi.org/10.1111/j.1475-6773.2010.01140.x

Rosenberg, M. (1956) 'Misanthropy and political ideology', *American Sociological Review*, 21(6), p 690. https://doi.org/10.2307/2088419

Ryan, M. (2020) 'In AI we trust: Ethics, artificial intelligence, and reliability', *Science and Engineering Ethics*, 26(5), pp 2749–67. https://doi.org/10.1007/s11948-020-00228-y

Ryan, S. et al (2020) *Understanding Experiences of Recruiting for, and Participating in, Genomics Research and Service Transformation: The 100,000 Genomes Project, 2015–17*, London: Policy Innovation and Evaluation Research Unit.

Sabat, I. et al (2020) 'United but divided: policy responses and people's perceptions in the EU during the COVID-19 outbreak', *Health Policy*, 124(9), pp 909–18. https://doi.org/10.1016/j.health pol.2020.06.009

Samuel, G. et al (2021) 'Ecologies of public trust: The NHS COVID-19 contact tracing app', *Journal of Bioethical Inquiry*, 18(4), pp 595–608. https://doi.org/10.1007/s11673-021-10127-x

Samuel, G. et al (2022) 'Public trust and trustworthiness in biobanking: the need for more reflexivity', *Biopreservation and Biobanking*, 20(3), pp 291-96. https://doi.org/10.1089/bio.2021.0109

Samuel, G.N. and Farsides, B. (2018a) 'Genomics England's implementation of its public engagement strategy: blurred boundaries between engagement for the United Kingdom's 100,000 Genomes project and the need for public support', *Public Understanding of Science*, 27(3), pp 352–64. https://doi.org/10.1177/0963662517747200

Samuel, G.N. and Farsides, B. (2018b) 'Public trust and "ethics review" as a commodity: the case of Genomics England Limited and the UK's 100,000 genomes project', *Medicine, Health Care and Philosophy*, 21(2), pp 159–68. https://doi.org/10.1007/s11 019-017-9810-1

Savage, N. (2016) 'Privacy: The myth of anonymity', *Nature*, 537, pp S70–S72. https://doi.org/10.1038/537S70a

Schaar, P. (2010) 'Privacy by design', *Identity in the Information Society*, 3(2), pp 267–74. https://doi.org/10.1007/s12394-010-0055-x

Schee, E. van der et al (2007) 'Public trust in health care: a comparison of Germany, The Netherlands, and England and Wales', *Health Policy*, 81(1), pp 56–67. https://doi.org/10.1016/j.healthpol.2006.04.004

Schee, E. van der (2016) *Public Trust in Health Care – Exploring the Mechanisms*. Available from: https://www.nivel.nl/sites/default/files/bestanden/Proefschrift_Public_trust_in_health_care_schee.pdf (Accessed: 12 July 2023).

Schee, E. van der, Jong, J.D. de and Groenewegen, P.P. (2012) 'The influence of a local, media covered hospital incident on public trust in health care', *European Journal of Public Health*, 22(4), pp 459–64. https://doi.org/10.1093/eurpub/ckr033

Schillinger, D., Chittamuru, D. and Ramírez, A.S. (2020) 'From "infodemics" to health promotion: a novel framework for the role of social media in public health', *American Journal of Public Health*, 110(9), pp 1393–6. https://doi.org/10.2105/AJPH.2020.305746

Schneider, P. (2005) 'Trust in micro-health insurance: an exploratory study in Rwanda', *Social Science & Medicine: Building Trust and Value in Health Systems in Low- and Middle-Income Countries*, 61(7), pp 1430–8. https://doi.org/10.1016/j.socscimed.2004.11.074

Schretzlmaier, P., Hecker, A. and Ammenwerth, E. (2022) 'Suitability of the Unified Theory of Acceptance and Use of Technology 2 Model for predicting mHealth acceptance using diabetes as an example: qualitative methods triangulation study', *JMIR Human Factors*, 9(1), p e34918. https://doi.org/10.2196/34918

Sedlakova, J. and Trachsel, M. (2022) 'Conversational artificial intelligence in psychotherapy: a new therapeutic tool or agent?', *The American Journal of Bioethics*, 23(5), pp 4–13. https://doi.org/10.1080/15265161.2022.2048739

Sekalala, S. et al (2020) 'Health and human rights are inextricably linked in the COVID-19 response', *BMJ Global Health*, 5(9), p e003359. https://doi.org/10.1136/bmjgh-2020-003359

Seligman, A.B. (1997) *The Problem of Trust*, Princeton: Princeton University Press.

Shahi, G.K., Dirkson, A. and Majchrzak, T.A. (2021) 'An exploratory study of COVID-19 misinformation on Twitter', *Online Social Networks and Media*, 22, p 100104. https://doi.org/10.1016/j.osnem.2020.100104

Shaw, D.M., Elger, B.S. and Colledge, F. (2014) 'What is a biobank? Differing definitions among biobank stakeholders', *Clinical Genetics*, 85(3), pp 223–7. https://doi.org/10.1111/cge.12268

Shaya, B. et al (2019) 'Factors associated with the public's trust in physicians in the context of the Lebanese healthcare system: a qualitative study', *BMC Health Services Research*, 19(1), p 525. https://doi.org/10.1186/s12913-019-4354-0

Shepherd, L., O'Carroll, R.E. and Ferguson, E. (2014) 'An international comparison of deceased and living organ donation/transplant rates in opt-in and opt-out systems: a panel study', *BMC Medicine*, 12: 131. https://doi.org/10.1186/s12916-014-0131-4

Shore, D.A. (2006) *The Trust Crisis in Healthcare: Causes, Consequences, and Cures,* New York: Oxford University Press. https://doi.org/10.1093/acprof:oso/9780195176360.001.0001

Sidani, S. et al (2010) 'Cultural adaptation and translation of measures: an integrated method', *Research in Nursing & Health*, 33(2), pp 133–43. https://doi.org/10.1002/nur.20364

Siegrist, M. and Bearth, A. (2021) 'Worldviews, trust, and risk perceptions shape public acceptance of COVID-19 public health measures', *Proceedings of the National Academy of Sciences*, 118(24), p e2100411118. https://doi.org/10.1073/pnas.2100411118

Silver, D. et al (2022) 'Association between COVID-19 vaccine hesitancy and trust in the medical profession and public health officials', *Preventive Medicine*, 164, p 107311. https://doi.org/10.1016/j.ypmed.2022.107311

Simpson, J.A. (2007) 'Psychological foundations of trust', *Current Directions in Psychological Science*, 16(5), pp 264–8. https://doi.org/10.1111/j.1467-8721.2007.00517.x

Smith, C. (2017) 'First, do no harm: institutional betrayal and trust in health care organizations', *Journal of Multidisciplinary Healthcare*, 10, pp 133–44. https://doi.org/10.2147/JMDH.S125885

Smith, S. et al (2005) Measurement of health-related quality of life for people with dementia: development of a new instrument (DEMQOL) and an evaluation of current methodology, *Health Technology Assessment*, 9(10). https://doi.org/10.3310/hta9100

Snyder, L.B. (2007) 'Health communication campaigns and their impact on behavior', *Diet and Communication*, 39(2, Supplement), pp S32–S40. https://doi.org/10.1016/j.jneb.2006.09.004

Solomon, S. and Abelson, J. (2012) 'Why and when should we use public deliberation?', *Hastings Center Report*, 42(2), pp 17–20. https://doi.org/10.1002/hast.27

Song, C. and Lee, J. (2016) 'Citizens' use of social media in government, perceived transparency, and trust in government', *Public Performance & Management Review*, 39(2), pp 430–53. https://doi.org/10.1080/15309576.2015.1108798

Stafford, I., Cole, A. and Heinz, D. (2022) *Analysing the Trust-Transparency Nexus: Multi-Level Governance in the UK, France and Germany*. Bristol: Policy Press.

Starke, G. (2021) 'The emperor's new clothes? Transparency and trust in machine learning for clinical neuroscience', in O. Friedrich et al (eds) *Clinical Neurotechnology meets Artificial Intelligence: Philosophical, Ethical, Legal and Social Implications*, Cham: Springer International Publishing, pp 183–96. https://doi.org/10.1007/978-3-030-64590-8_14

Starke, G. et al (2022) 'Intentional machines: a defence of trust in medical artificial intelligence', *Bioethics*, 36(2), pp 154–161. https://doi.org/10.1111/bioe.12891

Starke, G. and Ienca, M. (2022) 'Misplaced trust and distrust: how not to engage with medical artificial intelligence', *Cambridge Quarterly of Healthcare Ethics*, 20 October 2022 edn, pp 1–10. https://doi.org/10.1017/S0963180122000445

Stolle, D. (2015) 'Trusting strangers – the concept of generalized trust in perspective', *Austrian Journal of Political Science*, pp 397–412. Available from: https://nbn-resolving.org/urn:nbn:de:0168-ssoar-60076 (Accessed: 20 July 2023).

Straten, G.F.M., Friele, R.D. and Groenewegen, P.P. (2002) 'Public trust in Dutch health care', *Social Science & Medicine*, 55(2), pp 227–34. https://doi.org/10.1016/S0277-9536(01)00163-0

Streiner, D.L. and Norman, G.R. (2003) *Health Measurement Scales* (3rd edn), Oxford: Oxford University Press.

Suh, C.S., Chang, P.Y. and Lim, Y. (2012) 'Spill-up and spill-over of trust: an extended test of cultural and institutional theories of trust in South Korea', *Sociological Forum*, 27(2), pp 504–26. https://doi.org/10.1111/j.1573-7861.2012.01328.x

Sulik, J. et al (2021) 'Facing the pandemic with trust in science', *Humanities and Social Sciences Communications*, 8(1). https://doi.org/10.1057/s41599-021-00982-9

Šuriņa, S. et al (2021) 'Factors related to COVID-19 preventive behaviors: a structural equation model', *Frontiers in Psychology*, 12, p 676521. https://doi.org/10.3389/fpsyg.2021.676521

Swami, V. et al (2011) 'Conspiracist ideation in Britain and Austria: evidence of a monological belief system and associations between individual psychological differences and real-world and fictitious conspiracy theories', *British Journal of Psychology*, 102(3), pp 443–63. https://doi.org/10.1111/j.2044-8295.2010.02004.x

Sztompka, P. (1998) 'Trust, distrust and two paradoxes of democracy', *European Journal of Social Theory*, 1(1), pp 19–32. https://doi.org/10.1177/136843198001001003

Sztompka, P. (1999) *Trust: A Sociological Theory*. Cambridge: Cambridge University Press.

Tait, M. (2011) 'Trust and the public interest in the micropolitics of planning practice', *Journal of Planning Education and Research*, 31(2), pp 157–71. https://doi.org/10.1177/0739456X11402628

Tan, G.K.S. and Lim, S.S. (2022) 'Communicative strategies for building public confidence in data governance: analyzing Singapore's COVID-19 contact-tracing initiatives', *Big Data & Society*, 9(1), p 20539517221104090. https://doi.org/10.1177/20539517221104086

Taylor, L.A., Nong, P. and Platt, J. (2023) 'Fifty years of trust research in health care: a synthetic review', *The Milbank Quarterly*, 101(1), pp 126–78. https://doi.org/10.1111/1468-0009.12598

Thapa, C. and Camtepe, S. (2021) 'Precision health data: requirements, challenges and existing techniques for data security and privacy', *Computers in Biology and Medicine*, 129, p 104130. https://doi.org/10.1016/j.compbiomed.2020.104130

The European Social Survey European Research Infrastructure Consortium (2022) 'European Social Survey', [online]. Available from: https://www.europeansocialsurvey.org/ (Accessed: 20 October 2022).

Thomas, S.B. and Quinn, S.C. (1991) 'The Tuskegee Syphilis Study, 1932 to 1972: implications for HIV education and AIDS risk education programs in the black community', *American Journal of Public Health*, 81(11), pp 1498–1505. https://doi.org/10.2105/ajph.81.11.1498

Thorne, S.E. and Robinson, C.A. (1988) 'Reciprocal trust in health care relationships', *Journal of Advanced Nursing*, 13(6), pp 782–9. https://doi.org/10.1111/j.1365-2648.1988.tb00570.x

Told, M. (2022). Author conversation with Michaela Told about public trust and health diplomacy.

Tonković, M. et al (2021) 'Who believes in COVID-19 conspiracy theories in Croatia? Prevalence and predictors of conspiracy beliefs', *Frontiers in Psychology*, 12, p 643568. https://doi.org/10.3389/fpsyg.2021.643568

Topp, S.M. et al (2022) 'Building patient trust in health systems: a qualitative study of facework in the context of Aboriginal and Torres Strait Islander health workers' role in Queensland, Australia', *Social Science & Medicine*, 302, p 114984. https://doi.org/10.1016/j.socscimed.2022.114984

Topp, S.M. and Chipukuma, J.M. (2016) 'A qualitative study of the role of workplace and interpersonal trust in shaping service quality and responsiveness in Zambian primary health centres', *Health Policy and Planning*, 31(2), pp 192–204. https://doi.org/10.1093/heapol/czv041

Townsend, B. (2022) 'The lawful sharing of health research data in South Africa and beyond', *Information & Communications Technology Law*, 31(1), pp 17–34. https://doi.org/10.1080/13600834.2021.1918905

Turper, S. and Aarts, K. (2017) 'Political trust and sophistication: taking measurement seriously', *Social Indicators Research*, 130(1), pp 415–34. https://doi.org/10.1007/s11205-015-1182-4

Tutton, R., Kaye, J. and Hoeyer, K. (2004) 'Governing UK Biobank: the importance of ensuring public trust', *Trends in Biotechnology*, 22(6), pp 284–5. https://doi.org/10.1016/j.tibt ech.2004.04.007

United Nations (2020) *Global Cooperation Must Adapt to Meet Biggest Threat since Second World War, Secretary-General Says on International Day, as COVID-19 Transcends Border*, [online]. Available from: https://press.un.org/en/2020/sgsm20058.doc. htm (Accessed: 26 October 2022).

US Department of Health and Human Services FDA Center for Drug Evaluation and Research, US Department of Health and Human Services FDA Center for Biologics Evaluation and Research, and US Department of Health and Human Services FDA Center for Devices and Radiological Health (2006) 'Guidance for industry: patient-reported outcome measures: use in medical product development to support labeling claims: draft guidance', *Health and Quality of Life Outcomes*, 4, p 79. https://doi.org/ 10.1186/1477-7525-4-79

Van den Broucke, S. (2020) 'Why health promotion matters to the COVID-19 pandemic, and vice versa', *Health Promotion International*, 35(2), pp 181–6. https://doi.org/10.1093/heapro/daaa042

van der Meer, T.W.G. (2017) 'Political trust and the "crisis of democracy"', *Oxford Research Encyclopedia of Politics*, Oxford University Press. https://doi.org/10.1093/acrefore/9780190228 637.013.77

van Kessel, R. et al (2022) 'Digital health paradox: international policy perspectives to address increased health inequalities for people living with disabilities', *Journal of Medical Internet Research*, 24(2), p e33819. https://doi.org/10.2196/33819

Vayena, E. et al (2018) 'Digital health: meeting the ethical and policy challenges', *Swiss Medical Weekly*, 148(0304). https://doi.org/ 10.4414/smw.2018.14571

Vayena, E. and Blasimme, A. (2018) 'Health research with big data: time for systemic oversight', *The Journal of Law, Medicine & Ethics*, 46(1), pp 119-29. https://doi.org/10.1177/107311051 8766026

Verducci, S. and Schröer, A. (2010) 'Social trust', in H.K. Anheier and S. Toepler (eds) *International Encyclopedia of Civil Society*, New York, NY: Springer US, pp 1453–8. https://doi.org/10.1007/978-0-387-93996-4_68

Viskupič, F., Wiltse, D.L. and Meyer, B.A. (2022) Trust in physicians and trust in government predict COVID-19 vaccine uptake. *Social Science Quarterly*, 103(3), pp 509–520. https://doi.org/10.1111/ssqu.13147

Vollmer, S. et al (2018) 'Machine learning and AI research for Patient Benefit: 20 Critical Questions on Transparency, Replicability, Ethics and Effectiveness', [online]. Available from: http://arxiv.org/abs/1812.10404 (Accessed: 12 July 2023).

Vraga, E.K. and Bode, L. (2020) 'Defining misinformation and understanding its bounded nature: using expertise and evidence for describing misinformation', *Political Communication*, 37(1), pp 136–44. https://doi.org/10.1080/10584609.2020.1716500

Wang, D. and Mao, Z. (2021) 'A comparative study of public health and social measures of COVID-19 advocated in different countries', *Health Policy*, 125(8), pp 957–71. https://doi.org/10.1016/j.healthpol.2021.05.016

Wang, X., Shi, J. and Kong, H. (2021) 'Online health information seeking: a review and meta-analysis', *Health Communication*, 36(10), pp 1163–75. https://doi.org/10.1080/10410236.2020.1748829

Ward, P.R. et al (2015) 'A qualitative study of patient (dis)trust in public and private hospitals: the importance of choice and pragmatic acceptance for trust considerations in South Australia', *BMC Health Services Research*, 15(1), p 297. https://doi.org/10.1186/s12913-015-0967-0

Warkentin, M. et al (2002) 'Encouraging citizen adoption of e-Government by building trust', *Electronic Markets*, 12(3), pp 157–62. https://doi.org/10.1080/101967802320245929

Waszak, P.M., Kasprzycka-Waszak, W. and Kubanek, A. (2018) 'The spread of medical fake news in social media – The pilot quantitative study', *Health Policy and Technology*, 7(2), pp 115–18. https://doi.org/10.1016/j.hlpt.2018.03.002

Watson, N. and Halamka, J. (2006) 'Patients should have to opt out of national electronic care records', *BMJ*, 333(7557), pp 39–42. https://doi.org/10.1136/bmj.333.7557.39

Weatherford, M.S. (1992) 'Measuring political legitimacy', *American Political Science Review*, 2 September 2013 edn, 86(1), pp 149–66. https://doi.org/10.2307/1964021

Weber, G.M., Mandl, K.D. and Kohane, I.S. (2014) 'Finding the missing link for big biomedical data', *JAMA*, 311(24), pp 2479–80. https://doi.org/10.1001/jama.2014.4228

van der Weerd, W. et al (2011) 'Monitoring the level of government trust, risk perception and intention of the general public to adopt protective measures during the influenza A (H1N1) pandemic in the Netherlands', *BMC Public Health*, 11(1), p 575. https://doi.org/10.1186/1471-2458-11-575

Whetten, K. et al (2008) 'Trauma, mental health, distrust, and stigma among HIV-positive persons: implications for effective care', *Psychosomatic Medicine*, 70(5), pp 531–8. https://journals.lww.com/psychosomaticmedicine/Fulltext/2008/06000/Trauma,_Mental_Health,_Distrust,_and_Stigma_Among.3.aspx

White, S.K. (1990) *The Recent Work of Jürgen Habermas: Reason, Justice and Modernity,* Cambridge: Cambridge University Press.

Williams, G. and Fahy, N. (2019) 'Building and maintaining public trust to support the secondary use of personal health data', *Eurohealth*, 25(2), pp 7–10.

Wilson, M. (2005) *Constructing Measures*, London: Psychology Press.

Wood, M.J., Douglas, K.M. and Sutton, R.M. (2012) 'Dead and alive: beliefs in contradictory conspiracy theories', *Social Psychological and Personality Science*, 3(6), pp 767–73. https://doi.org/10.1177/1948550611434786

World Economic Forum (2022) 'Digital trust', [online]. Available from: https://www.weforum.org/projects/digital-trust (Accessed: 10 October 2022).

World Health Organization (2008) 'WHO outbreak communication planning guide', [online]. Available from: https://www.who.int/publications/i/item/9789241597449 (Accessed: 28 October 2022).

World Health Organization (2017a) 'Vaccination and trust – how concerns arise and the role of communication in mitigating crises', [online]. Available from: https://apps.who.int/iris/bitstream/han dle/10665/343299/WHO-EURO-2017-2908-42666-59448-eng.pdf?sequence=1&isAllowed=y (Accessed: 10 October 2022).

World Health Organization (2017b) 'WHO strategic framework for effective communications', [online]. Available from: https://cdn.who.int/media/docs/default-source/documents/commun ication-framework.pdf?sfvrsn=93aa6138_0 (Accessed: 21 October 2022).

World Health Organization (2019) 'Ten threats to global health in 2019', [online]. Available from: https://www.who.int/news-room/spotlight/ten-threats-to-global-health-in-2019 (Accessed: 6 May 2022).

World Health Organization (2020) *Immunization Agenda 2030: A Global Strategy to Leave No One Behind*, Geneva: WHO.

World Health Organization (2021) *Global Strategy on Digital Health 2020–2025*, Geneva: World Health Organization. Available from: https://apps.who.int/iris/handle/10665/344249 (Accessed: 15 May 2022).

World Health Organization (2022a) 'Toolkit for tackling misinformation on noncommunicable disease: forum for tackling misinformation on health and NCDs', [online]. Available from: https://apps.who.int/iris/rest/bitstreams/1474310/retri eve (Accessed: 20 July 2023).

World Health Organization (2022b) 'WHO coronavirus (COVID-19) dashboard', [online]. Available from: https://covid19.who.int/ (Accessed: 26 October 2022).

World Health Organization (2022c) 'WHO COVID-19 policy brief: building trust through risk communication and community engagement', [online]. Available from: https://apps.who.int/iris/rest/bitstreams/1465975/retrieve (Accessed: 20 October 2022).

World Health Organization (2023) 'WHO coronavirus (COVID-19) dashboard', [online]. Available from: https://covid19.who.int/ (Accessed: 19 July 2023).

World Health Organization Strategic Advisory Group of Experts (SAGE) on Immunization (2014) *Report of the Sage Working Group on Vaccine Hesitancy*, Geneva: WHO.

Xiong, X. et al (2021) 'Understanding public opinion regarding organ donation in China: a social media content analysis', *Science Progress*, 104(2), p 00368504211009665. https://doi.org/10.1177/00368504211009665

Yamanis, T., Nolan, E. and Shepler, S. (2016) 'Fears and misperceptions of the Ebola response system during the 2014–2015 outbreak in Sierra Leone', *PLOS Neglected Tropical Diseases*, 10(10), p e0005077. https://doi.org/10.1371/journal.pntd.0005077

Yang, S.-U., Kang, M. and Cha, H. (2015) 'A study on dialogic communication, trust, and distrust: testing a scale for measuring organization–public dialogic communication (OPDC)', *Journal of Public Relations Research*, 27(2), pp 175–92. https://doi.org/10.1080/1062726X.2015.1007998

Zhang, Z. and Min, X. (2020) 'The ethical dilemma of truth-telling in healthcare in China', *Journal of Bioethical Inquiry*, 17(3), pp 337–44. https://doi.org/10.1007/s11673-020-09979-6

Zhao, D., Zhao, H. and Cleary, P.D. (2019) 'Understanding the determinants of public trust in the health care system in China: an analysis of a cross-sectional survey', *Journal of Health Services Research & Policy*, 24(1), pp 37–43. https://doi.org/10.1177/1355819618799113

Index

References to tables and figures appear in **bold** type.